CLINICIAN'S GUIDE TO
VIOLENCE RISK ASSESSMENT

CLINICIAN'S GUIDE TO
VIOLENCE
RISK ASSESSMENT

Jeremy F. Mills
Daryl G. Kroner
Robert D. Morgan

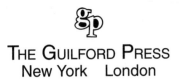

THE GUILFORD PRESS
New York   London

© 2011 The Guilford Press
A Division of Guilford Publications, Inc.
72 Spring Street, New York, NY 10012
www.guilford.com

Printed in the United States of America

This book is printed on acid-free paper.

Last digit is print number: 9 8 7 6 5 4 3 2 1

The authors have checked with sources believed to be reliable in their efforts to
provide information that is complete and generally in accord with the standards
of practice that are accepted at the time of publication. However, in view of the
possibility of human error or changes in behavioral, mental health, or medical
sciences, neither the authors, nor the editor and publisher, nor any other party
who has been involved in the preparation or publication of this work warrants
that the information contained herein is in every respect accurate or complete,
and they are not responsible for any errors or omissions or the results obtained
from the use of such information. Readers are encouraged to confirm the
information contained in this book with other sources.

Library of Congress Cataloging-in-Publication Data

Mills, Jeremy F.
  Clinician's guide to violence risk assessment / by Jeremy F. Mills, Daryl G. Kroner,
and Robert D. Morgan.
     p. cm.
  Includes bibliographical references and index.
  ISBN 978-1-60623-984-1 (hard cover : alk. paper)
  1. Violence—Risk assessment. 2. Violence. 3. Risk assessment.
I. Kroner, Daryl G.   II. Morgan, Robert D.   III. Title.
  RC569.5.V55M55 2011
  616.85′82075—dc22
                                                                    2010031636

ABOUT THE AUTHORS

Jeremy F. Mills, PhD, CPsych, is a psychologist with a practice in forensic, correctional, and counseling psychology in Kingston, Ontario, Canada. In addition, he serves as Adjunct Research Professor in the Department of Psychology at Carleton University in Ottawa. A Fellow of the American Psychological Association, Dr. Mills's research interests include violence risk assessment, violence risk communication, and the assessment of suicide risk. Dr. Mills provides consultation and training in the area of violence risk assessment.

Daryl G. Kroner, PhD, CPsych, is Assistant Professor in the Department of Criminology and Criminal Justice at Southern Illinois University Carbondale. Previously, he worked for 22 years as a prison psychologist. Dr. Kroner's research interests include correctional mental health, dynamic risk assessment during community supervision, and the social-context aspects of risk assessment.

Robert D. Morgan, PhD, is Associate Professor in the Department of Psychology at Texas Tech University in Lubbock, Texas. In addition, he is Director of Clinical and Forensic Services at Lubbock Regional Mental Health Mental Retardation Center. Dr. Morgan's research interests include correctional mental health, forensic psychology, and professional development and training.

PREFACE

This book is an applied and practical guide to the assessment of violence risk primarily for clinicians/practitioners or those learning to become clinicians. It should also prove helpful as an introduction for students and early-career professionals to the practical issues surrounding the clinical assessment of violence. We have found that the majority of clinicians who attend our risk assessment workshops are doctoral-level practitioners who have occasionally conducted violence risk assessments in their practice. This anecdotal observation was supported by a survey conducted by Tolman and Mullendore (2003), who found that although only 9% of clinical psychologists characterized their practices as forensic, 53% had conducted a risk assessment that was used in legal proceedings or criminal justice decision making, and 45% reported completing an assessment for criminal sentencing purposes. However, clinicians did not identify or rely on violence risk appraisal instruments in their assessments. Similarly, Nicholson and Norwood (2000) conducted a review of forensic assessments and concluded that assessors understood the legal question at hand, but they did not consistently use the assessment methods or instruments that had the strongest empirical basis for inclusion in the assessment process. Even among psychologists who specialize in forensic work, there is evidence of a reliance on less-than-optimal instruments in the assessment of risk for violence (Lally, 2003).

It is within this applied context that we have written this book to assist the clinician in making informed and scientifically supported assessments. We know that clinicians are pressed for time, so we have kept the historical references in the text to a minimum and focus primarily on what the current literature reflects, where the science of violence risk assessment seems to be going, what clinicians need to know to conduct risk assessments, and how to get started. We provide the reader with a broad array of risk appraisal instruments from various approaches and list publications that support their predictive validity. We are straightforward regarding our bias about how to conduct risk assessments and note differences from other perspectives where they exist. As practitioners on the front lines of a forensic practice where risk assessments are conducted routinely, we know the challenge of keeping up with the latest research and the importance of applying the best of forensic science to the assessment of violence.

To assist clinicians and students with limited experience in violence risk assessment, we have organized this book in a manner that coincides as much as possible with the assessment process, such that it can truly be used as a desk reference easily consulted for quick guidance. As a desk reference, this book is very practical in focus but based on current research, with more than enough references to provide any practitioner sufficient resource material to act as a competent expert witness if called to testify. We begin in Chapter 1 with an overview of the central issues, ethics, and risk factors that arise when assessing the risk for violence in adults. This overview is followed by a review of risk factors for various types of offenses in Chapter 2 and current risk assessment instruments for general, sexual, and spousal violence, including information on choosing appropriate instruments and their limitations, in Chapter 3. Chapter 4 reviews the conceptual issues and clinical dilemmas involved in violence risk assessment, and Chapter 5 presents an integrated–actuarial approach to assessment and management of violence risk. We conclude with a review of the assessment process in Chapter 6 and a step-by-step discussion of report writing in Chapter 7.

In the headlong search to improve the assessment of violence risk and improve public safety, perhaps at times we inadvertently come to believe that dangerous people can be identified and that harm can always be avoided. David Carson (2008) suggests that clinicians in the risk assessment enterprise need to adopt precepts or "self-evident truths" (p. 141) that pertain to risk assessment. Among these precepts are that risk is a part of life and harm will sometimes occur, that the occurrence of harm does not mean that a poor risk decision was made, that risk assessment relies on imperfect knowledge, and that risk management functions with finite resources. These precepts are necessary to ground ourselves in the reality of what we undertake when we conduct a risk assessment. Sometimes, in spite of our best efforts, harm still occurs. However, in the assessment of violence risk, only our best effort will do.

ACKNOWLEDGMENTS

We are grateful to Catherine Serna-McDonald, Christopher Romani, and Andrew Gray for reviewing drafts of this manuscript.

CONTENTS

CLINICIAN'S GUIDE TO
VIOLENCE RISK ASSESSMENT

CHAPTER 1

■ ■ ■

VIOLENCE RISK ASSESSMENT

An Introduction

For a variety of purposes, and in a range of settings, clinicians may be involved in providing formal assessments for the courts or other quasi-judicial boards. In fact some estimates have shown that approximately half of all psychologists in general practice will at some point provide an assessment for the court (Tolman & Mullendore, 2003). Although readers of this clinician's guide are likely to be interested in the practice of violence risk assessment, the assessment and management of violence risk is not limited to forensic psychologists and psychiatrists. Approximately 25% of offenders will seek community-based mental health services (Morgan, Rozycki, & Wilson, 2004); thus, the

> assessment and management of violence risk are critical issues, not just for psychologists and psychiatrists in forensic settings but for all practicing clinicians. Despite a long-standing controversy about the ability of mental health professionals to predict violence, the courts continue to rely on them for advice on these issues and in many cases have imposed on them a legal duty to take action when they know or should know that a patient poses a risk of serious danger to others. (Borum, 1996, p. 954)

To ensure consistency of terminology between us as writers and you as readers, we define our use of the term *risk assessment*. Many times in the literature the term "risk assessment" refers to the determination of the level of risk (risk estimation), whether actuarial (percent likelihood) or descriptive (low, moderate, or high). When we refer to risk assessment we are referring to the whole process of (1) determining an individual's level of risk (risk

1

estimation), (2) identifying the salient risk factors that contribute to that risk, (3) identifying risk management strategies and considerations to manage or minimize that risk, and (4) communicating the risk information to the decision maker.

This book will lead you through the practical steps of conducting one type of clinical assessment, a violence risk assessment. Violence risk assessments are almost always completed within the context of the competing interests of society (public safety) and the person being assessed (freedom and fairness). Clinicians typically form a therapeutic alliance with their clients, working jointly to improve their lives. However, within the violence risk assessment process, we emphasize a reliance on the *data* (the specific facts as they relate to the potential for violence) to avoid therapeutic bias. The forensic assessor is partial to neither "side" in a legal proceeding, but to whatever conclusions and recommendations to which the facts and case specifics point. It therefore follows that forensic assessments of violence risk will differ from other clinical assessments in approach, content, and tenor. For example, a clinical assessment is typically conducted to aid in the rehabilitation of the client, whereas a forensic (violence) assessment typically aids in answering a legal question, with the focus of protecting society at large. These differences also lead to what appear to be competing ethical obligations not typically experienced within clinical practice.

In this opening chapter we introduce you to some of the issues surrounding violence risk assessment. The information we provide assumes a certain level of training and experience and so we have adopted the term *clinician* as we understand that similar training and experience may be found in different disciplines (psychology, psychiatry, nursing, social work, etc.). In outlining some of the essential skills the clinician needs to bring to the process, we will identify *who* should be conducting a violence risk assessment. Clinicians are often asked to provide an opinion regarding the potential for violence of a client. There are competing arguments for and against conducting these types of assessments. We review some of these arguments to answer the question of *why* a clinician should undertake a violence risk assessment.

As a clinician you are very familiar with therapeutic reports and assessments, but we introduce you to some of the similarities and differences between therapeutic assessments and violence risk assessments. Differences between these two types of assessments include differences in the scope, purpose, procedures, and reports. We also review the advances that have been made in violence risk assessment over the past few decades to set our approach within the development of the field and to demonstrate that it represents the current direction of violence risk assessment. From a historical perspective, violence risk assessment has moved from purely clinical judgment of dangerousness to an actuarial approach with reliance on probabilities based on statistical information. We show that over time actuarial measures have been combined with dynamic risk factors within a risk management and intervention paradigm, resulting in what we term an *integrated–actuarial* approach. We also report on an emerging approach that integrates changes in dynamic risk factors that modify static–actuarial estimates and is now in the forefront of violence risk assessment. We refer to this approach as a *dynamic–actuarial* approach. With our review of the differences between therapeutic and violence risk assessment and the overview of assessment advances we hope to introduce *what* a violence risk assessment should include. Finally, we look at the special ethical obligations that are associated with conducting violence risk assessments. The purpose of ethical standards is to ensure that *how* we conduct violence risk assessments meets the highest standards of science and professional practice.

THE CLINICIAN'S KNOWLEDGE AND TRAINING

The purpose of this book is to provide knowledge on the specifics of violence risk assessment for professionals who already provide other types of clinical intervention and assessment services. *Clinician* is the term we have chosen to describe those professionals who have advanced knowledge and training in a number of areas important for the conducting of violence risk assessment. This knowledge and training is not specific to any particular professional group but can be found in psychology, psychiatry, psychiatric nursing, counseling, and social work. It is the clinician's ethical responsi-

---

Actuarial Risk Assessment

The term *actuarial* means "relating to statistical calculation" (Merriam-Webster's Collegiate Dictionary, 1999). Confusion exists within the literature because some researchers have equated instruments that are primarily composed of static and historical risk factors with the term actuarial. In fact, instruments with potentially changeable factors can and do incorporate actuarial risk estimates. Also, actuarial has sometimes been used to describe instruments that are not "structured clinical/professional judgment." So to be clear, *actuarial* is a term we reserve for any instrument that has a structured scoring method and associates a statistical or probabilistic statement with the resulting score. To run the risk of complicating things further, instruments that employ the structured professional judgment (more on this later in the chapter) approaches could quite easily become "actuarial" simply by applying statistical probabilities to the resulting scores. While this would be, in our opinion, an improvement, it is not in keeping with the structured professional judgment approach to risk assessment.

bility to judge if he or she is competent to complete a violence risk assessment. Most professional governing bodies will have specific guidance on what would constitute competence. Similarly we assume that clinicians will belong to a licensing body that regulates their profession through standards of practice and ethical guidelines. In keeping with this we are assuming that the clinician will operate within these guidelines.

Violence risk assessment requires graduate-level training or equivalent knowledge and experience in understanding personality and psychopathology. Similar levels of knowledge and training are necessary in the areas of theories of behavior and interviewing skills. Experience and competence in the area of case formulation and clinical report writing are very important. A comprehensive knowledge of mental and personality disorders and their relationship to behavior in general and violence in particular are essential. While it is not necessary to be able to diagnose a mental disorder, in many cases it is essential to have access to a professional who can diagnose a mental disorder and/or personality disorder, as these disorders are features of some risk appraisal instruments. Finally, knowledge of statistics and an ability to apply and communicate their meaning in an assessment context is also important. Terms such as *receiver operating characteristic* and *base rates*, although cumbersome to some, are essential for analyzing and communicating the results of risk assessments.

A Word about Statistics

Clinicians often dislike statistics. However, we are making the assumption that you may have to testify in court and may be called upon to express an opinion based upon the scientific literature. The relationship of risk appraisal instruments with violence will be featured prominently throughout this book, and to that end we have included enough statistical information for you to speak to the issue of risk assessment.

Researchers employ many different types of statistics in order to communicate the accuracy of a given risk appraisal instrument. Among these statistics is the more commonly known and understood Pearson's r (between two continuous variables), point–biserial correlation (between continuous and dichotomous variables), or phi coefficient (which is a measure of the degree of association between two binary variables). Other statistics used include percent correct classifications, relative improvement over chance (RIOC), positive predictive power (which is the proportion of those predicted to fail who actually did fail), Cohen's d, and area under the curve (AUC) from a receiver operating characteristic (ROC), among many others.

For ease of understanding we will report correlation statistics and AUC statistics. The latter statistic is a relatively recent development but is appealing because of its robustness as a statistical measure of accuracy and ease of understanding for lay consumers of information. ROC analysis has its origins in signal-detection theory in engineering and psychophysics (Green & Swets, 1966; Swets, 1988). Research by Marnie Rice and Grant Harris (1995, 2005) has helped to promote the more frequent use of ROC and make it better understood within forensic contexts. AUCs can be interpreted as the probability that a randomly selected recidivist will have a higher score than a randomly selected nonrecidivist. For example, most AUCs fall within the range of .50 (chance) to 1.0 (perfect prediction). If an instrument used to predict recidivism had an associated AUC of .75, this means that there is a 75% likelihood that the score of a randomly selected recidivist would be higher than the score of a randomly selected nonrecidivist. Conceptually this is easier to explain than other types of statistics. From an accuracy perspective the AUC is not as susceptible to changes in the *base rate* (the sample mean likelihood for an outcome) as are measures of correlation. As an example, point–biserial correlations of .100, .243, and .371 are considered small, medium, and large, respectively, when the base rate (overall likelihood of recidivism) is 50% (see Harris & Rice, 2005). These correspond to AUCs of .556, .639, and .714 for small, medium, and large effect sizes. If the base rate for recidivism changes to 25%, then point–biserial correlations of .086, .212, and .327 would correspondingly be considered low, medium, and high. A more complete listing of equivalent values between AUC, Cohen's *d*, and point–biserial correlations is reported by Rice and Harris (2005).

Another illustration of the correlation versus ROC difference was the result of a statistical exercise by one of us (JM). Using previously published data, a known predictor of recidivism was correlated with the dichotomous outcome of recidivism (point–biserial correlation) which resulted in a moderate and significant correlation. The data were then manipulated so that recidivism failure was indicated only for the top scorers so that the AUC would equal 1.0, perfect prediction. A point–biserial correlation was then undertaken on the manipulated data and resulted in a correlation approximating $r = .82$. This illustrates that when point–biserial correlations are reported in recidivism studies they do not have the same theoretical range of −1.0 to +1.0 as would potentially be the case when two truly continuous variables are correlated.

WHY CONDUCT VIOLENCE RISK ASSESSMENTS?

The arguments for and against conducting violence risk assessments are at times addressed under cross-examination. Thus, a basic understanding of these arguments may assist a clinician in giving testimony. In addition, these arguments help to outline how a local criminal justice agency can benefit from a rational, empirically based, routine violence risk assessment. In this section, we review common reasons for conducting violence risk assessments, along with some criticisms of risk assessment.

Public Safety

The tension between the autonomy of the client and an obligation to protect foreseeable victims from a client's violent actions was central to the *Tarasoff v. Regents of the University of California* (1976) decision. This decision continues to have a significant role in current ethical standards, legal decisions, and lawmaking that governs mental health services. Embedded in this decision is the requirement to assess clients for potential violence. Even if a clinician never plans to do forensic work, at some point he or she may be required to conduct an assessment and act on the conclusion. Therefore, every clinician needs to be competent to assess risk for potential violence (most jurisdictions in the United States and Canada have endorsed the *Tarasoff* duty-to-protect decision, and de facto a requirement to assess). But just what kind of assessment is required of a clinician, particularly one who is not working formally as a forensic psychologist?

The *Tarasoff* decision gives a broad legal requirement for clinicians to assess for specific or targeted violence. There is a duty to protect that stems from the *Tarasoff* findings when the clinician has reasonable grounds to believe a specific individual is at imminent risk of serious harm or death. Clinicians should be aware that the criteria for the duty to protect may vary somewhat by jurisdiction due to legal interpretations and professional standards of practice. Additionally, they should be aware of the impact that these specific guidelines will have on their practices.

The focus of this book is on the longer term assessment of violence risk, not on *Tarasoff* situations. In general there are five significant differences between conducting a longer term violence risk assessment and determining the duty to protect in a *Tarasoff* situation. First, "duty-to-protect" arises when you are treating a client. Violence risk assessments, on the other hand, typically happen outside the context of treatment. Second, the clinician has a choice whether to conduct a formal violence risk assessment. The clinician in these situations selects assessment methods, management strategies, and instruments, and considers base rates and placing risk within a context. Conversely, in treatment, when a clinician determines that a client may pose a clear risk to another person, the clinician has no choice but to conduct a *Tarasoff* evaluation. Third, *Tarasoff* situations generally occur when a specific person (or group of persons) can be identified as being at risk for violence by the client, whereas longer term violence risk assessments more often focus on the risk to society in general. Fourth, *Tarasoff* situations typically focus on imminent risk as opposed to long-term risk. (Imminence, though, may arise when conducting a long-term violence risk assessment, at which time one is then required to conduct a *Tarasoff* evaluation, notify appropriate authorities and the potential victim, and include the evaluation in the broader violence risk assessment report.)

Fifth, the strategies for conducting a *Tarasoff* assessment are different from the strategies for conducting a violence risk assessment. Borum and Reddy (2001) argue that the *Tarasoff* assessment is more deductive and relies more upon clinical judgment as compared to violence risk assessments, which focus on a broad array of risk factors and base rates. They use the acronym ACTION to outline the areas for consideration in a *Tarasoff* evaluation: Attitudes supportive of violence, Capacity to carry out the threat, Thresholds crossed in a progression of behavior, Intent to act versus threats alone, Other's knowledge of the client, and Non-compliance with strategies to reduce risk. We reiterate that it is very important for the clinician to have a clear understanding of the local jurisdiction's requirements surrounding the duty to protect.

While *Tarasoff* introduces the legal obligation for therapists to consider pubic safety, we believe clinicians have a broader duty to public safety through violence risk assessment. Applying a validated assessment protocol systematically in cases requiring violence risk assessments will more consistently identify high-risk offenders over unstructured decision making (Nugent, 2000). That improved consistency has the potential to reduce violence because it will lead to the detention, treatment, and management of high-risk cases, with the result of improved public safety. Informed decisions based on valid risk assessment instruments will provide better decisions than those based on no assessment, and in most cases better than clinical judgment alone (Hilton & Simmons, 2001). In addition, a risk assessment will be able to suggest evidence-based strategies that may reduce the likelihood of future violence. Decision makers can then use these suggestions in forming their dispositions.

Increased Fairness for the Client

Balancing public safety and the assessed person's rights is one outcome of conducting ethical, competent violence risk assessments. In order to contribute to this balance, the clinician must have a strong commitment to present findings in keeping with the facts of the case (the data), rather than advocating for either the assessed person or those representing public safety. The best approach to balancing this tension is to "conduct objective risk evaluations according to the best standards available" (Tolman & Rotzien, 2007, p. 73).

In addition to presenting findings in keeping with the facts, there are specific ways to facilitate a better balance between public safety and the client's rights. For example, the inclusion of a standardized violence risk assessment may increase the potential for a fair decision for the assessed person by reducing the relative influence of other factors not related to risk. Some of these factors include public pressure, fears and emotions of the decision maker, the influence of the last case (recency effect), and prejudices stemming from ignorance such as overestimating the risk posed by the mentally ill. The clinician who can present an assessed person's risk within a context (e.g., compare the client's probabilities with other relevant probabilities, or explain the psychosocial contributors or mental health contributors to the behavior) will give the decision maker a better basis on which to make a decision. Courts and boards of review are the arbiters of the public interest and weigh the rights of the assessed person with the protection of society. A properly conducted violence risk assessment can provide such decision makers with a broader picture, such as describing how the assessed person could have his or her level of risk reduced or managed. With that broader context in hand, the decision maker could then determine that release is possible, despite the potential for future violence. For example, release destinations (halfway houses, inpatient units, etc.) often differ in levels of services available, whether they are for supervision or intervention and treatment. If your report identifies supports and supervision that can be put in place to help an assessed person avoid violent behavior, it may give a decision maker confidence in releasing the assessed person, rather than detaining him or her further.

Value-Added Information for Decision Makers

The research into violence risk factors has increased our knowledge on the risk factors among diverse samples. With the current risk assessment literature, clinicians can better account for individual differences among assessed persons. Standardizing individual differences is an important advancement in the risk assessment enterprise. For example, psychopathy has been shown to have predictive value with sexual offenders (Olver & Wong, 2006): the higher a person scores on a psychopathy scale, the more likely he or she is to commit a future sex offense. Other research has shown that including deviant arousal with psychopathy improved the prediction of sexual recidivism (Harris et al., 2003). This result has also been found with juvenile sexual offenders (Gretton, McBride, Hare, O'Shaughnessy, & Kumka, 2001). Factoring in these kinds of individual differences allows clinicians to provide more reliable and precise risk assessments, thereby providing more information on risk factors and the potential intervention and management associated with those risk factors to the decision makers.

Arguments against Risk Assessment

Despite the general acceptance of violence risk assessment, there are some who have argued against conducting them. Campbell (2000) likened the use of clinical judgment and guided clinical risk assessment (what we call structured professional judgment)[1] to phrenology (personality assessment based upon the shape of the individual's head) in terms of meeting the requirements for admissibility in court. He further suggested that there was no known error rate for these methods, and therefore they did not meet the *Daubert* criteria for admissibility of scientific evidence in court (*Daubert v. Merrell Dow Pharmaceuticals*, 1993). Although the *Daubert* ruling did not provide a checklist for admissibility of scientific information, it did outline several guidelines: (1) the theories and techniques used in the assessment process need to be falsifiable, (2) the techniques must have a known error rate, (3) the method used has to have been subjected to peer review and publication, and (4) the method used has to have found widespread acceptance in the relevant scientific community. In a subsequent paper, Campbell (2003) took issue with the classification errors of actuarial risk assessments and concluded that psychologists undertaking such assessment had to accept that they offered "very limited accuracy" (p. 277).[2] Despite these objections, Tolman and Rogzien (2007) note that not all states follow the *Daubert* criteria, that the Supreme Court has stated the necessity of expert testimony in assessing violence potential (*Addison v. Texas*, 1979), and that research has found that actuarial data are admissible in court over 90% of the time (Tolman & Rhodes, 2005). The courts' general acceptance of actuarial data seems the undoing of these arguments of admissibility.

Another criticism of conducting risk assessments relates to the generalization of risk assessment to specific groups of offenders (Whiteacre, 2006). For example, despite a number of studies that have shown a significant relationship between the actuarial risk instrument, the Level of Service Inventory—Revised, and women offenders' recidivism (see Chapter 3), the use of this instrument with women offenders has drawn some criticism (Holtfreter & Cupp. 2007). Some of the criticisms appear to be rooted in ideology (feminist "pathways to crime" vs. a gender-neutral social learning theory), while other concerns have more merit and are empirically based. It is true that many of the instruments developed with men offenders have not been as extensively researched with women offenders, yet evidence for their validity remains. In recent years a growing emphasis on the unique issues and needs of women offenders suggests that this discrepancy in risk assessment instrument evaluation will be resolved with time and more research (Blanchette & Brown, 2006). It is also quite likely that some risk factors that effectively predict violence with men may not predict as well with women, or the manner in which risk factors are measured may need to be

---

[1]Later in this chapter we cover in some detail the different approaches to risk assessment.

[2]Without getting ahead of ourselves, actuarial estimates assume a degree of error. More will be said on this later.

adjusted to accommodate gender differences. These differences do not mean risk assessment should be abandoned, but rather that we need to adjust risk assessment protocols to accommodate these differences. In fact, examples of risk appraisal instruments that have been modified to account for differences between adult and juvenile offenders include the Level of Service Inventory—Revised and the Psychopathy Checklist—Revised (Youth Level of Service/Case Management Inventory 2.0 and Psychopathy Checklist—Youth Version, respectively).[3]

Some researchers are looking empirically at both gender-neutral and gender-responsive risk factors with the aim of improving assessment accuracy. Wright, Salisbury, and Van Voorhis (2007) examined both of these types of risk factors as they relate to incarcerated women offenders and their subsequent institutional misconduct and found that both types of variables were related to misconduct. The strength of the relationship with misconduct was very similar for both types of risk factors, leading these researchers to conclude that there is room for both risk factors when assessing women offenders.

In any case, having a competent violence risk assessment, even if it does not account for group-specific differences, will be better than having none at all. We also note that limitations of the assessment based upon these differences do need to be clearly stated. Hilton and Simmons (2001) provide an excellent example of what contributes to risk decisions when actuarial data are ignored. In their study, a tribunal board made decisions to detain or to transfer forensic psychiatric patients to lower security. The variables examined included patient characteristics, patient history, clinical presentation, and the actuarial risk estimates of the Violence Risk Appraisal Guide (VRAG). Compared to other variables, the senior clinician's testimony was the strongest predictor of the tribunal's decisions. What, then, predicted the senior clinician's decisions? They were (1) institutional management problems, (2) psychotropic medication use and success, (3) the patient's physical attractiveness, and (4) the patient's preindex criminal history. The actuarial risk estimates as measured by the VRAG were not related to the tribunal decision ($r(169) = .06$), team recommendation ($r(160) = .01$), or the senior clinician testimony ($r(152) = -.02$). Essentially, the attractiveness of the patient was more of a factor in the decisions than the actuarial risk estimates. This is disappointing and somewhat surprising, given that the VRAG was developed at the institution where the study was conducted.

In our opinion the benefits of public safety and improved decision making for both society and the assessed person outweigh the limitations that

---

[3]Similar adjustments have also been undertaken in psychology more broadly when considering the measure of intelligence or psychopathology.

are evident in the violence risk assessment process. Clinicians need to be aware of the differences between risk assessment and clinical assessment, the current practice in risk assessment, and the ethical considerations when undertaking risk assessment in order for the benefits to be realized. These issues are the topics covered in the next sections.

THERAPEUTIC VERSUS VIOLENCE RISK ASSESSMENTS

As we have noted, we assume that the clinician brings to the violence risk assessment knowledge and experience in conducting a clinical assessment and writing a therapeutic report. However, therapeutic clinical assessments differ from violence risk assessments (see also Heilbrun, Marczyk, Dematteo, & Mack-Allen, 2007) and clinicians should not assume that clinical skills alone are sufficient. As noted by Skeem and Golding (1998), "Occasionally experts rely primarily on their traditional clinical skills and attempt to generalize these to psycholegal assessment" (p. 365). Even with solid clinical training, clinicians need to understand the basic and unique characteristics of conducting violence risk assessments before they agree to undertake the task. Understanding these conceptual differences will (1) assist in providing a focus and purposeful framework for conducting risk assessments, (2) highlight aspects of clinical training that contrast with conducting a risk assessment, and (3) reduce the likelihood of applying procedures for therapeutic assessments to violence risk assessments inappropriately. Traditional clinical therapeutic assessment and the violence risk assessment share some common features, but are also different in key ways. These differences have to do with the scope of the work, the importance of the assessed person's perspective, voluntariness, autonomy, threats to validity, and the nature of the assessor–client relationship.

Similarities between Therapeutic Assessments and Violence Risk Assessments

Both therapeutic assessments and violence risk assessments require a reasonable degree of scientific certainty. For example, according to the ethical code of the American Psychological Association, "Psychologists' work is based upon established scientific and professional knowledge of the discipline" (2.04). Other mental health disciplines share similar expectations. Thus, in both the therapeutic and violence risk assessment, clinicians must be able to justify their techniques, conclusions, opinions, and recommendations. With both kinds of assessment there will be a merging of scientific theories and procedures with training and experience.

No assessment includes all information. It simply is not possible in a therapeutic or violence risk assessment to obtain all information. Rather, the goal is to obtain as much relevant information as is reasonable to secure and necessary to answer the referral question ethically and scientifically. Both therapeutic and violence risk assessment results must be presented in an accurate, organized, and easily understood format. The therapeutic assessment and violence risk assessment will both present similar types of information. In fact, certain components of the assessment reports overlap. As one example, a psychosocial history will be common to both types of assessment. Finally, competent assessment techniques are, naturally, a necessity for both the therapeutic assessor and the violence risk assessor.

Differences between Therapeutic and Violence Risk Assessments

Despite the similarities between therapeutic and violence risk assessments, there are important differences between them.[4] Generally, the scope and focus of the therapeutic assessment is broad and tends to be geared toward identifying and understanding psychopathology for the purpose of guiding interventions. However, the therapeutic assessment is more likely to involve multiple contacts with the patient. The violence risk assessment, on the other hand, is very specific with the predetermined goal of predicting future behavior, and is typically limited to one or two contacts.

The purpose of the therapeutic assessment is to aid in the rehabilitation of a patient. Although the guidelines for this type of assessment are predominantly standards of practice, this is not to say that a therapeutic assessment is void of legal standards. In fact, standards of practice for therapeutic assessment are influenced by legal decisions. The violence risk assessment, however, presents a unique shift for the clinical generalist, one that includes the recognition that the client is not necessarily the individual being assessed. Because the client in a violence risk assessment may not be the person being assessed we try to use the term *assessed person*. Furthermore, a violence risk assessment is requested to help answer a legal question that is before a legally constituted decision-making body (e.g., court, forensic mental health board, parole board). The legal question in these instances is often to what degree the assessed person poses a threat of violence to others. Thus, the guidelines for conducting a violence risk assessment are likely to involve both a legal standard (i.e., meeting standards for admissibility to

---

[4]Interested readers are referred to Heilbrun, Marczyk, DeMatteo, and Mack-Allen (2007); Melton et al. (2007); Packer (2008); and Skeem and Golding (1998) for a more thorough review of the differences between therapeutic assessments and violence risk assessments.

court proceedings) as well as standards of practice by a governing body (i.e., licensing board).

Astute and ethical clinicians recognize these differences between the therapeutic assessment and the violence risk assessment and develop their procedures accordingly, beginning with the initial contact. The initial contact outlines the assessment process, with explicit reference to a third party. In fact, licensing boards may require both a written and a verbal notification of both parties' involvement in the assessment. The therapeutic assessment focuses on the collection of treatment-relevant information concerning a patient's daily functioning, mental status, and identification of psychopathology. The client is generally assumed to be credible, since in a treatment context there are fewer motives to withhold or distort information. Although clients in therapeutic assessments are prone to subconscious distortions, there is generally less intent to deceive or manipulate the assessor. Reliability and validity of psychological tests (e.g., MMPI2, WAIS-IV) are not the primary foci, as accuracy is secondary to understanding the client's perspective. For example, exaggerated responses on a psychometric test have a different set of implications within a therapeutic setting (where there may well be a cry for help) than within a violence risk assessment (where it's more likely an interviewee is malingering for gain). The person being assessed in a violence risk assessment may consciously and intentionally distort information (e.g., present in an overly favorable manner). Thus, the reliability and validity of assessment information are of great importance, and clinicians need to take special care to assess for dissimulation. Furthermore, the procedures used to address the referral question are generally not scrutinized in many therapeutic settings, whereas the procedures used to assess the risk for violence are often carefully scrutinized, sometimes under cross-examination in a court room.

The time frame of the therapeutic assessment is generally determined by client need (e.g., severity of condition), and may be more leisurely paced. The schedule for a violence risk assessment, on the other hand, is often predetermined by the governing body and is therefore outside of the clinician's control. The client requesting a violence risk assessment may require a quick response time, or may be in no particular hurry, so there may be significant differences in time frames to complete the evaluation.

The report for a therapeutic assessment is written in technical language, is read by other health professionals, and contains diagnostic formulations (i.e., DSM language). Psychological and psychiatric terms are often included, and the tone of the report may be caring, empathic, and nurturing, with an emphasis on trust and confidentiality. The structure of the report is often left to the discretion of the psychologist, with the content of the report generally limited to issues and information of therapeutic relevance.

In contrast, the report for a violence risk assessment is read by lawyers, judges, and releasing bodies, and contains information relevant to all legal issues pertinent to the case. Issues surrounding the limits to confidentiality become more complex. In fact, we recommend that the report explicitly state such limits and how consent, with regard to these limits, was obtained. The structure of the report is often determined by the legal issue at hand as there are frequently multiple stages of the legal question that need to be systematically covered in a report. Psychological jargon has no place in a violence risk assessment. Instead, plain and professional language should be employed, with care taken to explain technical terms. The primary reason for this approach is that the consumers of the violence risk assessment are typically not clinicians and are generally not familiar with the acronyms and technical terms utilized by those who work within the mental health arena.

With a therapeutic assessment, the client is likely to be a voluntary participant, and the clinician will have autonomy in addressing the clinical issues, usually with the cooperation of and input from the client. Violence risk assessments, on the other hand, are generally requested by a third party (e.g., court or decision-making body) such that the individual being assessed typically has little choice as to whether the assessment is completed. In fact, even if the individual refuses to participate in the assessment process, in some jurisdictions a report with the clinician's opinions will be provided to the governing body requesting the violence risk assessment. In such circumstances the clinician's opinion, based on other available information, is still considered in the decision-making process. In these situations, the assessed person's choice is limited to whether he or she will choose to participate in the assessment process.

With therapeutic assessments the assessor in most clinical situations has clear ethical duties to respect the dignity of and provide responsible care for the client. The clinician is operating with substantial therapeutic responsibilities, and therefore developing a working alliance is critical for success. The clinician is generally working on behalf of the patient. However, within a violence risk assessment, the assessed person may have no helping alliance with the assessor. The main responsibility is to the decision-making body, with a focus on documentation. Moreover, the assessed person may or may not find the content within the report helpful to his or her current situation (Packer, 2008).[5]

These differences between clinical and violence risk assessments outline

---

[5]Although there may be no formal alliance with the assessed person, rapport remains a valued goal as the more effort the assessor puts into establishing a relationship with the individual being assessed, the greater the likelihood for a more fully informed assessment. More specifically, efforts should be taken to foster an accepting and empathic attitude with the individual; the mere purpose of a violence risk assessment does not warrant a callous and distant interpersonal interaction.

part of the challenge of conducting an assessment within the forensic arena. We turn next to a brief history of the advances in violence risk assessment over the past decades. Understanding these advances will help you understand how the field has reached the current practice and where the field is likely to go in the coming years. It will also set our recommended approach within the historical context of risk assessment.

ADVANCEMENTS IN RISK ASSESSMENT

Assessing "dangerousness" has for many years represented the intersection between the legal system and the mental health system (Monahan, 1984). In fact, *dangerousness* is more of a legal term than a meaningful mental health construct. It has been suggested that for advancements to occur in risk assessments, research must first distinguish among the component parts of dangerousness: risk factors (the variables that predict violence), harm (the degree of violence), and risk (the likelihood of violence) (Steadman et al., 1994). Through the years research has focused on risk factors and on risk likelihood, but less so on the assessment-of-harm component.

Advancements in risk assessment have been described as "generational" by different authors (Andrews, Bonta, & Wormith, 2006; Doyle & Dolan, 2002). These descriptions seem to be tied to the advent of specific risk assessment tools as opposed to paradigm shifts. Doyle and Dolan accounted for advancements as moving from clinical judgment (first-generation risk assessments), to actuarial judgments (second-generation risk assessments), and then to currently structured clinical/professional judgment (third-generation risk assessments). Later Andrews, Bonta, and Wormith identified clinical judgment as first generation in which they included structured clinical judgment. They then identified empirically based but atheoretical instruments as second generation and then empirically based instruments that included static and dynamic factors as third generation. They proposed a fourth generation that "guides and follows service and supervision from intake through case closure" (p. 8). Our recapitulation of the advancements in risk assessment (see Figure 1.1) is focused more on the approach to the overall assessment process and less on specific instruments, though clearly one is associated with the other.

Clinical Judgment of Risk

The authority of the clinical judgment estimate of risk relies solely upon the clinician's subjective evaluation of the case factors. There are no formal rules or guidelines to identify risk factors and no specifications on how to integrate identified risk factors. There are no decision-making guidelines in

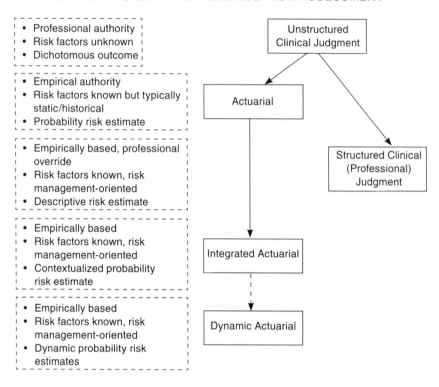

FIGURE 1.1. Advancements in risk assessment.

terms of what constitutes elevated risk, and there is no integration of the base rate (average rate) of violence. Clinical judgment is inaccurate mainly because it fails to systematically consider empirically based risk factors. Even if those risk factors are known and assessed by the clinician, the integration of the information is inconsistent. Research into decision making in other areas has shown that both laypersons and professionals fail to incorporate multiple pieces of information into their decisions (Northcraft & Neale, 1987; in a poststudy analysis only the amateurs knew they were influenced by a single piece of information whereas the professionals had more confidence that they had considered many sources of information). In addition to being unable to integrate multiple pieces of information systematically, individuals tend to make decisions without considering the base rate of the outcome (Kahneman & Tversky, 1973).

Moreover, clinicians are not immune to influences of the graphic nature or severity of violence, and may be unduly influenced by the context in which the assessment takes place, the clinician's personal characteristics, and the personal characteristics of the offender (Hilton & Simmons, 2001;

Static and Dynamic Risk Factors

Static risk factors are those risk factors that are related to the outcome (crime, violence, sexual violence, etc.) but do not change over time. These would include age of first offense or prior history of alcohol abuse. Some static risk factors can change over the long term but are called static because they generally do not change between the time of the assessment and the point of a new conviction. Example of these types of risk factors can include number of prior incarcerations and number of prior violent offenses.

Dynamic risk factors are those risk factors that are related to the outcome that have the potential to change over time. These risk factors have sometimes been referred to as "criminogenic need areas" (see Andrews & Bonta, 2010)—areas of functioning (attitudes, associates, substance abuse, etc.) that are related to outcome but can be potentially changed by appropriate intervention. In most instances within the literature when researchers report on dynamic risk factors they are really reporting on *potentially* dynamic risk factors. A truly dynamic risk factor is one that is empirically shown to change over time and that change over time must be related to a change in the likelihood of the outcome (risk). In fact this strict application of dynamic has been rarely demonstrated within the literature on risk assessment.

Hilton, Harris, Rawson, & Beach, 2005). Further, clinical judgment often involves backward inference (deriving causal links from historical information that is known in the present). The clinician has much latitude in identifying past facts to explain the behavior but this does not always mean those prior facts were indeed causal. For example, knowing that psychosis is related to violence (relatively small contribution) and that the person assessed who was violent also suffered from schizophrenia would lead some clinicians to conclude (infer) that the person was violent because of his or her mental illness and therefore will be violent in the future because of his or her mental illness. However, other clinicians who understood that research has found that mental illness is infrequently related to crime in the mentally ill (Junginger, Claypoole, Laygo, & Cristanti, 2006) may not infer the same causal relationship and arrive at a very different conclusion.

Because of the influences of backward inference, variable knowledge of risk factors, and personal characteristics of the offender on subjective judgment, agreement among forensic clinicians tends to be low. Stated another way, the accuracy of a measure (in this case the clinical judgment) cannot exceed the reliability of the measurements (in this case the ability for agreement in assessment). For example, think of a ruler with fuzzy lines and numbers. Two different people use the ruler to measure the same distance. The accuracy of the distance measurement (validity) cannot exceed the ability of each of those two people to agree on the distance (reliability). A ruler with sharply focused lines is more likely to produce the same measurement when used by more than one person. Clinical judgments lack accuracy because they inconsistently measure risk factors. As evidence accumulated that clinical judgment was not an accurate way to predict violence, alternate methods began to appear (Monahan, 1983, 1996).

Actuarial Assessment

Advocacy for an actuarial risk estimate for use in parole decision making is not new. Hornell Hart recommended that the Parole Board of Massachusetts utilize "prognostic scores" (p. 410) associated with probabilities of parole failure as far back as 1923. In addition to individual research efforts that have shown actuarial assessment to be more accurate than clinical assessment when predicting general violence (Harris, Rice, & Cormier, 2002) and sexual violence (Bengtson & Langstrom, 2007), meta-analyses consistently favor actuarial over clinical (subjective) decision making. Grove and Meehl (1996) considered a broad array of decisions across many disciplines (e.g., bankruptcy, parole violation, adjustment to the military), and found actuarial methods to be more accurate overall than subjective methods.[6] Additionally, meta-analytic results demonstrate the superiority of statistical (actuarial) assessment over clinical assessment among sex offenders (Hanson & Bussiere, 1998).

In a recent meta-analysis by Hanson and Morton-Bourgon (2009), the data showed actuarial assessments of sex offender risk to be more accurate than structured professional (clinical) judgment. In a separate meta-analysis, in which clinician decision making was specifically identified, the data showed that actuarial assessments continued to perform better than clinician judgments (Aegisdottir et al., 2006). Actuarial approaches to risk classification can be as simple as scoring a person's criminal history (e.g., scoring the Static-99, a sexual violence actuarial instrument), or as complex as making sophisticated iterative classification tree analyses requiring computer support (Banks et al., 2004). Actuarial risk instruments have been shown to increase in predictive accuracy when scored with high reliability, when items are not missing, and when individuals within the samples have the same opportunity (time) to reoffend (Harris & Rice, 2003).

Actuarial instruments tend to be robust across groups of offenders. Dennis Doren (2004) compared the original risk estimates of two actuarial measures, the Static-99 (Hanson & Thornton, 2000) and the Rapid Risk

---

[6]These authors found 136 suitable studies in which actuarial systems performed better in 64 studies, there were mixed results in another 64 studies, and clinical judgment performed better in eight studies.

Meta-Analysis

Meta-analysis is a relatively new statistical method, which has grown in use over the past 15 years, of combining the findings from multiple research studies to determine what the overall effect size (strength of relationship) might be between a predictor variable and an outcome variable. The formulas for combing the findings can become quite complicated as correlations, chi-squares, and t-tests must all be mathematically changed to a common metric, usually r or Cohen's d. The strength of meta-analysis is the ability to compare different variables from across studies as they relate to the outcome of interest. A weakness is that many of the studies must be collapsed into common variables, and this sometimes leads to combining variables that are not measuring the same construct. Overall, a methodologically sound meta-analysis can provide much information into the relative importance of variables across a wide variety of settings.

Assessment for Sex Offence Recidivism (Hanson, 1997), with risk estimates from a combined group of studies that differed from the original samples on which the instruments were developed. This was undertaken to determine if the original risk estimates generalized to other samples of sexual offenders. Generally the results were positive, indicating fairly consistent risk estimates; however, there were some discrepancies particularly with the Static-99. When the comparison studies were examined individually there was a general finding that risk estimates were more aligned with the original estimates for samples that shared a similar base rate and follow-up time. A similar base rate simply means that the offenders were similar in terms of their overall risk level. Another unreported and related contributor to differences would also include the distribution of the offenders' risk scores. For example, a sample with a low base rate (lower average risk) is likely to have fewer individuals with higher scores. If the sample has fewer individuals with high scores, then the resulting risk estimates for those high scorers will be *unstable* because the group of high scorers is too small a sample. Those who are opposed to actuarial risk assessment may use these types of findings to bring disrepute on the process when in fact the explanation is not so much process but weak statistical comparisons.

Actuarial risk assessment accepts error in the ability to predict violence in at least three ways. First, it acknowledges that the world is inherently uncertain.[7] Second, it permits determinism at the level of the physical world, but believes that our knowledge of that world will always be fragmentary

---

[7] Actuarial estimates reflect the premise that the world is inherently uncertain and, regardless of how much information is available, certainty is not possible.

and imperfect. Third, it accepts that the use of an equation or algorithm can never capture the richness and full complexity of the phenomenon it is meant to predict. Actuarial assessment also demands empirical evidence rather than professional authority as the source of predictive validity.

There are some limitations to a purely actuarial approach to risk assessment. First, actuarial instruments tend to focus on historical or static risk factors, and there has been a tendency for the scores only to change to indicate more risk. For example, the number of prior violent offenses is a static risk factor (it will not change between the time of the assessment and the next possible offense), but over the long term the individual may commit more violent offenses and this risk factor may worsen. Second, these static factors tend to provide little information about the specific areas that should be targeted for intervention. For example, knowing the age of first violent offense is an excellent predictor but offers little information on the treatment targets for intervention. Third, actuarial instruments provide estimates of risk, and there is a need to cross-validate the instruments on different populations of individuals to ensure predictive accuracy. This may not be as much of a limitation as some detractors would suggest, given that intelligence and personality measures are often adjusted for different populations when measuring specific constructs. Fourth, static risk factors often do not suggest an etiology for the behavior they predict, which is often a question of inquiry when assessments are conducted. Fifth, actuarial methods become less accurate when predicting increasingly rarer events; as the base rate of a behavior decreases, so does the accuracy of actuarial estimates (though one would argue the same for clinical judgment, structured or otherwise).

Dawes, Faust, and Meehl (1989) suggested that professionals continue to ignore the advantage of actuarial over clinical judgment decisions due to habit or misconception based on training, theoretical understanding, or personal values. They debunk a common argument that group statistics do not apply to single individuals or events by suggesting that this position overlooks the fact that it is the common features shared among persons that permits *any* prediction of behavior. Much of clinical hypothesizing of future behavior is predicated on the observation of factors that would indicate the likelihood of the behavior. Extrapolation of individuals' responses to psychometric testing to current or subsequent behavior/experiences is predicated on relating individual responses to group norms. The clinical integration of this information, however, is not transparent, as it happened within the confines of the clinician's head—and we would argue is unique in each instance a judgment is made. The clinical process (the exact factors and method of combining those factors) cannot be measured and therefore tested empirically. Actuarial methods, by contrast, are transparent; they can be tested and they can be critiqued. Dawes et al. (1989) concluded that "failure to accept a large and consistent body of scientific evidence over unvalidated personal observation may be described as a normal human failing or, in the case of professionals who identify themselves as scientific, plainly irrational" (p. 1673).

Structured Professional (Clinical) Judgment

Structured Professional Judgment (SPJ) is a process that identifies and rates a number of risk factors as clearly not present, may be present, or definitely present. Examples of SPJ instruments include the HCR-20 (Webster, Douglas, Eaves, & Hart, 1997), which is used to predict general violence in correctional and forensic settings; the Spousal Assault Risk Assessment (SARA; Kropp, Hart, Webster, & Eaves, 1994), for spouse assault; and the SVR-20 (Boer, Hart, Kropp, & Webster, 1997), for sexual violence.

Proponents of SPJ advocate in favor of a risk management or violence prevention model over a purely actuarial approach (Douglas & Kropp, 2002). This SPJ approach identifies the salient risk factors through the use of structured scoring. These risk factors include both static and dynamic variables. Based upon the number of risk factors present and the subjective importance of specific risk factors to the assessor, the assessor makes a judgment as to the risk an individual represents (low, moderate, or high). This method imposes a structure on the evaluation and sets as a minimum the number of risk factors to be considered through the use of the SPJ instrument. Following the identification of the risk factors, the clinician makes suggestions on how best to intervene to reduce risk or how best to manage the risk the individual poses.

SPJ differs from purely clinical judgment in that risk factors are reliably identified and integrated for an overall classification of risk. SPJ differs primarily from purely actuarial assessment in that it does not offer a probability statement. Some have referred to SPJ as "ostensibly a moderate position but in fact clinical judgment in new clothing" (Hilton, Harris, & Rice, 2006). The strength of this approach is the structure imposed on measuring the risk factors and the focus on risk management.

The SPJ approach has the clinician assess the structured risk factors from the specific instrument (usually 20), incorporate other risk factors or weight some risk factors with greater weight than others, and then make a determination of risk (typically characterizing risk as low, moderate, or high). The central limitations to the SPJ method are the absence of numerical probabilities and the allowance for clinical override in the estimate of risk: that is, the adjustment of the estimate by the assessor based upon other risk factors. Hanson and Morton-Bourgon (2009) reviewed three studies that reported an actuarial risk score and an adjusted actuarial risk rating. Raters (correctional staff) within these studies were permitted to adjust the final risk rating of an actuarial instrument based upon other factors. In each case the adjusted risk ratings were not as accurate as the actuarial risk score. With evidence that base rates are not routinely incorporated in clinical risk appraisal, and that descriptive categories tend to be perceived by both clinician and laypersons as being of greater risk than actuarially supported for acts of violence, we see it as an important step to anchor risk assessment with an actuarially determined probabilistic statement wherever possible. In a nutshell, what advocates of SPJ view as a strength (the ability to incorporate or weight additional information at the clinician's discretion), we view as a weakness. We see this process of override as a return to clinical judgment.

Integrated–Actuarial Risk Assessment

Among the criticisms of purely actuarial risk assessment was that the approach omitted from consideration pertinent risk factors not captured by the actuarially based instruments. Other criticisms painted actuarial assessment as void of dynamic risk factors, intervention recommendations, and risk management strategies. Further, criticisms pointed to the absence of "critical" risk factors, those deemed particularly germane to the case. In many respects this argument was a straw man used by some advocates of SPJ who prefer to use descriptive categories and clinical override over an actuarially anchored assessment. In response to these criticisms of purely actuarial risk assessments, experts have advocated for the inclusion of both actuarial information and risk management strategies within risk assessment (Dvoskin & Heilbrun, 2001; Heilbrun, Dvoskin, Hart, & McNiel, 1999). Since the early 1990s we have been conducting actuarially based violence risk assessments, and we have never written an assessment without including comments on intervention recommendations and risk management strategies. In order to distinguish between a purely actuarial assessment as has been represented in some of the literature from what we have been practicing for many years, we have employed the term *integrated–actuarial risk assessment* to refer to the integration of (1) actuarial risk estimates, with (2) potentially dynamic risk factors, (3) intervention/treatment recommendations, and (4) risk management strategies within the overall risk assessment process.

Dynamic–Actuarial Risk Assessment

We have coined the term *dynamic–actuarial risk assessment* to refer to risk assessment procedures that measure both static and dynamic factors and that in the remeasurement of those dynamic factors can potentially alter the actuarial estimate of an individual's risk (Mills, 2005). This is unique as it potentially changes actuarial risk estimates through reassessment of risk factors. Note that research in the field on this approach is still very much at the beginnings of development—with some room for optimism but no replicated applied findings at this point.

Harris and Rice (2003) correctly note that the measurement of any construct at a single point in time is a static measure. Researchers often refer to dynamic variables (e.g., antisocial attitudes, criminal associates, alcohol use) or items in a scale as "dynamic" when what is meant is that those items are potentially changeable. Whether or not the risk factors are dynamic is an empirical question, as is whether or not the change is meaningfully related to risk. It is also important to note that researchers will sometimes add potentially dynamic variables (attitudes, mood, etc.) to static/historical variables in an attempt to demonstrate that dynamic variables can add to the prediction of recidivism over static information alone. The question that so often goes unanswered is whether it is the content of the construct versus a change in the construct that is contributing to the improved prediction. More often than not it is the former that is being demonstrated and not the latter.

Having said this, the focus of researchers who are on the cutting edge of the risk assessment field is to identify a reliable and theoretically relevant measure that can account for actual change in risk to reoffend. These measures include both static/historical and potentially changeable or dynamic items. The *dynamic–actuarial risk assessment* measures dynamic items repeatedly whereas the static/historical items are measured only once.

The Violence Risk Scale (VRS; Wong & Gordon, 2006) is a more recently peer-reviewed instrument that was specifically developed to assess change in risk that may occur during the treatment of violent offenders and also measures how much change the treatment has produced. The VRS contains 20 dynamic variables and only 6 static variables. Correlations with violent recidivism varied by length of follow-up but were significant for both the static (r = .21 to .31) and dynamic (r = .28 to .40) variables. Presently, no peer-reviewed research has been identified that demonstrates changes in the VRS scores to be related to recidivism; however, one retrospective study using a sex offender version showed some success in this regard (Olver, Wong, Nicholaichuk, & Gordon, 2007). This provides reason for optimism that as research continues more dynamic measures of risk will be available to the clinician.

Perhaps the closest risk appraisal instrument to a truly dynamic–actuarial risk assessment is the combination of the Static-99, Stable-2007, and Acute-2007—a combination that forms the Dynamic Supervision Project (Hanson, Harris, Scott, & Helmus, 2007). With this assessment process, the initial static assessment of risk can be adjusted by changes to the dynamic risk factors, which are measured repeatedly over time during the offender's postrelease in the community. (We'll say more about this project in the next chapter.)

At this point in the development of the field, we advocate for the integration of dynamic and actuarial information that will, first, establish an underlying level of actuarial risk; second, inform that risk from an etiological perspective; third, suggest risk management strategies that reflect the integration of both actuarial and dynamic risk factors; and fourth, communicate the risk information to decision makers effectively.[8] Underlying all of these procedures is the clinician's commitment to ethical practice. We view ethics not so much as a list of rules, but rather as guidelines that will ensure scientifically sound, fair, and thorough risk assessments that can benefit both society and the assessed person. We next look at these ethical guidelines, which though specific to psychology should be accepted practice by any clinician undertaking the risk assessment process.

ETHICS ESSENTIALS

Ethical Practice and Violence Risk Assessment

Clinicians must comply with standards of ethical practice. For example, psychologists are obligated to comply with the *Ethical Principles of Psychologists and Code of Conduct* (American Psychological Association, 2002). However, in no other arena are the principles of ethical practice more prominent than in forensic assessment, including violence risk assessment. In a study of ethical dilemmas, Pope and Vetter (1992) discovered that forensic psychology ranked fifth out of 23 categories of practice for reported ethical concerns. Personal liberties are typically at risk when clients are evaluated for risk of future violent behavior, and we submit that clinicians engaged in the assessment of risk should be held to an especially high ethical standard. In fact, the uniqueness of forensic work, including violence risk assessment, necessitates specialty guidelines and principles of ethical practice. The *Specialty Guidelines for Forensic Psychologists* (1991) was developed by the Committee on Ethical Guidelines for Forensic Psychologists of the American Psychological Association. Whether you are an experienced clinician with thousands of evaluations under your belt, or a neophyte clinician, we encourage you to reread your specific profession's code of conduct as well as your licensing board rules and regulations. In Table 1.1 we highlight the

---

[8]We are by no means the first to recommend the integration of risk estimation and risk management. Some have done so in an attempt at resolving the conflict in the literature between advocates of actuarial risk estimation and clinical risk determination (Dvoskin & Heilbrun, 2001), others because the science of violence prediction was pointing them in that direction (Hanson & Harris, 2000; Hanson, Harris, Scott, & Helmus, 2007; Thornton, 2005), and still others because of the need to measure risk-related treatment change (Olver, Wong, Nicholaichuk, & Gordon, 2007; Wong & Gordon, 2006).

standards and guidelines from our respective codes (i.e., *Ethical Principles of Psychologists and Code of Conduct* [American Psychological Association], 2002]; *Specialty Guidelines for Forensic Psychologists* [Committee on Ethical Guidelines for Forensic Psychologists, 1991]) most applicable in the assessment of risk for violence.

When reviewing Table 1.1 we suggest you read the guidelines and answer the question, "Do I meet this standard of practice?" For example, Guideline III notes the following "provides services only in areas in which they have specialized knowledge, skill, experience, and education." In the far right column we have provided space where you can note for self-evaluation purposes whether you meet the criteria. This exercise will give you an opportunity to identify areas of practice that requires further training, knowledge, or supervision in order for you to provide high-quality violence risk assessment.

Ethical Pitfalls in Violence Risk Assessment

A common pitfall in clinical practice is the use of techniques without proper training (Caudill, 2002). This is particularly applicable when discussing actuarial risk assessment and SPJ models of risk assessment. We contend that clinicians who perform risk assessments but do not keep abreast of developments in the field of violence risk assessment are practicing unethically. To be current, one simply must keep up with debates about the use of actuarial risk assessments with or without professional overrides, proposed advantages of SPJ, statistical concepts that are directly relevant to risk assessment, such as base rates, and other developments in the field. Books such as this one as well as attendance at workshops and symposia will assist in keeping you current. As noted in both the *Ethical Principles of Psychologists and Code of Conduct* (American Psychological Association, 2002) and the *Specialty Guidelines for Forensic Psychologists* (Committee on Ethical Guidelines for Forensic Psychologists, 1991), it is the psychologist's responsibility to ensure that he or she is *competent* to provide the services offered, and this includes competence in the techniques utilized within his or her work. Other mental health professions (e.g., psychiatry, social work) have comparable ethical codes of conduct.

Other pitfalls in psychological assessment that appear relevant for violence risk assessment include confirmation bias, unstandardizing tests, and ignoring the effects of low base rates (Pope, 2003). According to Pope, confirmation bias occurs when we give undue weight to data that support our initial opinions and hypotheses, resulting in a "premature cognitive commitment" to our initial impressions (see Chapter 6, "The Risk Assessment Process," for discussion of avoiding the confirmation bias in violence risk assessment). Unstandardizing tests includes changing administration

(*text continues on page 30*)

TABLE 1.1. Summary of Ethical Guidelines Relevant for the Provision of Violence Risk Assessments

Ethical standard	Ethical Principles of Psychologists and Code of Conduct (American Psychological Association, 2002)	Specialty Guidelines for Forensic Psychologists (Committee on Ethical Guidelines for Forensic Psychologists, 1991)	Criteria met/ not met
Responsibility	• Psychologists are aware of their professional and scientific responsibilities to society and to the specific communities in which they provide risk assessment services. (Principle B: Fidelity and Responsibility)	Guideline II. Responsibility. Forensic psychologists: • Provide risk assessments in a manner that is consistent with the highest standards of the profession. • Make a reasonable effort to ensure that the results/opinions of the risk assessment are used in a forthright and responsible manner.	
Competence	• Psychologists must be qualified by education, training, or experience to provide risk assessments and use risk assessment techniques, e.g., actuarial measures. (Standard 2.01)	Guideline III. Competence. Forensic psychologists: • Provide services only in areas in which they have specialized knowledge, skill, experience, and education. • Present to the client (e.g., Court) the boundaries of their competence, the factual bases for their qualifications, and relevance of those qualifications to the risk of violence. • Are responsible for knowledge and understanding of the legal and professional standards which govern their forensic practice. • Are obligated to understand and uphold the civil rights of the offenders they assess. Recognize their personal values, moral beliefs, or personal/professional relationships that may interfere with competent performance of their risk assessment.	
Relationships	• Avoid multiple relationships (e.g., treating an offender and then asked to complete a violence risk assessment). (Standard 3.05) • Obtain the *informed consent* of individuals using language that is reasonably understandable to that person or persons. (Standard 3.10)	Guideline IV. Relationships. Forensic psychologists: • Inform the client of factors that might reasonably affect the decision to contract with the examiner for purposes of completing a risk assessment. • Do not provide risk assessments on the basis of contingent fees when the service includes expert testimony or the provision of affirmations or representations relied upon by third parties.	

(continued)

- Should offer a portion of risk assessment services on a pro bono or reduced fee basis when public interest or welfare of clients may be inhibited by limited resources.
- Recognize and seek to minimize dual role relationships.
- Ensure informed consent to include the client's legal rights, purposes of the risk assessment, nature of the evaluation, intended use of results, and who employed the examiner.
- Inform legal authorities of sources of conflict between the psychologist's professional standards and requirements of legal standards.

Guideline VI. Methods and Procedures. Forensic psychologists:

- Maintain current knowledge of scientific, professional and legal developments within the area of violence risk assessments ... use that knowledge, consistent with accepted clinical and scientific standards, in selecting data collection methods and procedures for the evaluation.
- Make available all data that form the basis for their evidence or risk assessment evaluation.
- Avoid undue influence upon their methods, procedures, and products of risk assessment resulting from financial compensation or other gains.
- Do not complete risk assessments on individuals not adequately represented by legal counsel.
- Seek data/records from third parties only with prior approval of the relevant legal party.
- Are aware of hearsay exceptions and other rules governing expert testimony.
- Have an affirmative duty to ensure that their written products and oral testimony conform to the Federal Rules of Procedure (12.2[c]) or its state equivalence.

- Psychologists are responsible for ensuring that informed consent was attained. (Standard 3.10)
- Offenders must be informed of the nature, purpose, and uses of evaluation even if they refuse to participate. (Standard 3.10)

Assessment

- Use techniques sufficient to substantiate your findings. (Standard 9.01)
- Provide opinions only after conducting an evaluation of an individual (attempt to see them in person for purposes of your risk assessment and rely on file reviews or collaterals only when offenders will not participate in the evaluation). (Standard 9.01)
- Use tests for their designed purpose and in the designed manner (in light of the research). (Standard 9.02)
- Use tests that are reliable and valid. (Standard 9.02)
- Use tests that are language appropriate. (Standard 9.02)
- Release raw test data to qualified professionals if release permits it. Test data includes "raw and scaled scores, client/patient responses to test questions or stimuli, and psychologists' notes and recordings concerning client/patient statements and behavior during examinations." (Standard 9.04)

TABLE 1.1. (*continued*)

Ethical standard	*Ethical Principles of Psychologists and Code of Conduct* (American Psychological Association, 2002)	*Specialty Guidelines for Forensic Psychologists* (Committee on Ethical Guidelines for Forensic Psychologists, 1991)	Criteria met/ not met
	• Use current tests, strategies/techniques. (Standard 9.08) • Psychologists are responsible for protecting the integrity and security of all test materials including test manuals, instruments, protocols, and test questions/stimuli. (Standard 9.11)		
Confidentiality	• Psychologists have a primary obligation to take reasonable precautions to protect confidential information obtained during the course of a risk assessment evaluation while recognizing that limits to confidentiality exist. (Standard 4.01) • Psychologists discuss with offenders the limits on confidentiality regarding the results of the risk assessment. (Standard 4.02) • When consulting with colleagues regarding a risk assessment, psychologists do not disclose confidential information and disclose information only to the extent necessary to achieve the purpose of the consultation. (Standard 4.06)	Guideline V. Confidentiality and Privilege. Forensic psychologists: • Are aware of legal standards that may affect or limit confidentiality or privilege attached to the risk assessment. • Inform clients of the limitations to the confidentiality of the risk assessment. • Make every effort to maintain confidentiality with regard to any information that does not bear directly upon the legal purpose of the risk assessment. • Provide clients access to information and results of the risk assessment with a meaningful explanation of the information.	

| Communications | • Psychologists are responsible for the accuracy of the results, even if those results are obtained from test scoring and interpretation services. (Standard 9.09) | Guideline VII. Public and Professional Communications. Forensic psychologists:
• Make reasonable efforts that results of their risk assessment are communicated in ways that will promote understanding and avoid deception.
• Ordinarily avoid making detailed public statements about a violent risk prediction.
• Have an obligation to all parties when testifying in legal proceeding to present their risk assessment findings, conclusions, evidence, or other professional products in a fair manner.
• Actively disclose all sources of information utilized in a risk assessment.
• Are aware that their essential role as expert to the court is to assist the trier of fact to understand the evidence or to determine a fact in the prediction of violence risk. |

instructions, test items, or scoring procedures (i.e., such that the test is no longer truly standardized). Ignoring the effects of low base rates (lower base rates are present in the prediction of sexual and violence risk over general recidivism risk) will result in misclassifying many offenders as violent. As noted above, Mills et al. (2010) found that clinicians lack understanding of base rates as they pertain to risk for future violent behavior and, more important, overestimate the likelihood of violence risk.

In addition to these common pitfalls, there are other potential blind-spots unique to the ethical practice of forensic mental health:

• *Promising too much.* Many clinicians encounter this pitfall unintentionally. Many clinicians enter the field because of a desire to help others, and it is this desire to be helpful that can unwittingly lead to promises that exceed what one can offer. This seems an easy pitfall to avoid: even early career clinicians know that they should not promise an opinion before an assessment is conducted. However, it is easier to be caught in a situation of promising to provide a service he or she is not qualified to perform. For example, you may agree to conduct a violence risk assessment only to learn that one of the issues to be assessed is risk for fire setting, which is a unique outcome that very few could attest they have expertise in assessing. Thus, although it may seem obvious, clinicians must never promise an outcome. Limit the guarantees you give to the specific type of evaluation you will conduct; the nature of the report you will submit to the attorney, court, or parole board; and the expected time frame for completion of the evaluation and report.

• *Substituting advocacy for scientific objectivity.* When conducting any forensic evaluation, including assessment of violence risk, accuracy takes precedence over understanding or appreciating the assessed person's view and recommending what may be in his or her best interest (Goldstein, 2003). The critical issue is for forensic examiners to recognize their role in providing accurate assessments of risk for future violent behavior, regardless of their personal beliefs or attitudes toward an assessed person.

• *Letting values overshadow empirically based findings.* Forensic examiners cannot allow their personal values and beliefs to interfere with the assessment process. For example, if you are requested to conduct a risk assessment for future violent behavior in the criminal sentencing phase of a capital murder trial, any beliefs you have about the death penalty cannot interfere with your evaluation or the opinions you provide to the court. We all have our biases; however, it is your ethical responsibility to ensure that your biases do not impede your assessment or color the results and the opinions you put forth. It is better to decline an assessment if you suspect your biases or personal beliefs may enter into the assessment process.

• *Doing a cursory job.* Violence risk assessment requires substantial time. Clinicians involved in this line of professional service should commit themselves to the time necessary to complete a comprehensive evaluation. It is not uncommon, in our experience, for a thorough risk assessment to require 20 or more hours of work by the time one has read previous investigative reports, interviewed collateral informants, and conducted assessment and testing procedures. Doing a cursory job and providing opinions based on an evaluation that is not thorough contradicts ethical obligations of forensic psychologists, including the guidelines for using appropriate methods and procedures ("maintain professional integrity by examining the issues at hand from all reasonable perspectives, actively seeking information"; Committee on Ethical Guidelines for Forensic Psychologists, 1991).

Dual Roles as an Ethical Pitfall in Violence Risk Assessments

The issue of dual roles is sufficiently important and in our experience occurs frequently enough to warrant additional elaboration as a potential ethical pitfall. A common question presented to professionals involved in violence risk assessment is whether clinicians can ethically provide forensic treatment and conduct a violence risk assessment with the same person. It is optimal, in multistaff settings or where specialized resources are available, that the treatment and assessment reporting responsibilities be separated. A conflict can readily arise for a clinician who conducts a violence risk assessment *after* providing treatment because the therapeutic alliance the clinician has formed with the assessed person will make it hard for him or her to remain objective. Even when the assessment is conducted first, a conflict can arise because the clinician is going to be remunerated for the subsequent treatment. Clearly dual-role conflicts need to be avoided wherever possible.

When logistics or resources prohibit a separation of treatment from assessment roles (i.e., when dual roles are unavoidable, such as in correctional or forensic facilities with one clinician), clinicians need to take explicit steps to reduce potential conflict. It is the clinician's ethical obligation to cause no harm and minimize the negative consequences where dual relationships are unavoidable. Further, it is imperative that the multiple responsibilities that stem from dual roles be communicated to the assessed person as part of the informed consent process. For example, if a clinician providing therapy may later have to provide a report on how successfully that therapy addressed the issue of violence, then this needs to be explicitly stated ahead of time, before treatment begins. Multiple roles and responsibilities are often unavoidable and are professionally and ethically appropriate when there is no viable alternative and when the clinician understands and prepares for them (Heltzel, 2007).

Examples from general and criminal justice-oriented clinical arenas illustrate how difficult it can be to serve dual roles, but also how it is feasible. *Tarasoff* issues present a prime example from general (noncriminal justice) clinical practice. Since the *Tarasoff* ruling, it is clear that clinicians involved in the provision of therapeutic services have a responsibility to assess when a client poses a risk for harm to others. When a clinician conducts an assessment in a criminal justice setting, he or she usually has multiple responsibilities, which may include ensuring the personal safety of the client (such as suicide potential), ensuring public safety (such as disclosure of escape plans), actual treatment, and conducting assessments for a variety of purposes. Not every assessment situation will require the clinician to pay attention to all these possible responsibilities, but the clinician needs to be aware of the potential for conflicting roles (and allegiances), and ensure that he or she is fulfilling these roles. Given that the list of responsibilities for clinicians continues to expand, the best practice (legally and ethically) is to formulate risk assessment endeavors not according to roles, but according to responsibilities. Doing so will make it clear how you separate your work as a therapist from your work as a forensic evaluator. The primary responsibility when conducting a violence risk assessment is to make it thorough and objective.

CONCLUSION

This chapter introduced you to a specific type of clinical assessment: the violence risk assessment. We assume the clinician brings with him or her an understanding of general clinical practice and the obligation to professional standards, knowledge, competency, and ethical practice. We have covered in general terms why violence risk assessments are conducted. This enterprise is not without controversy, but we hope to have demonstrated that there is an important and arguably an essential role for the clinician in the assessment of violence risk. We have introduced the difference between clinical/ therapeutic assessments and violence risk assessment and the advances in risk assessments over the past several decades. Advances in risk assessment continue, so clinicians can expect the "state of the art" to change over time—which is all the more reason to remain current in the field when risk assessment is a part of your practice. Finally, we provided you the opportunity to assess your own readiness for violence risk assessment through a review of the ethical standards of practice. The next chapter examines the risk factors associated with different specific violent outcomes.

CHAPTER 2

■ ■ ■

VIOLENCE RISK FACTORS

Our focus in this book is on general violence assessment, which typically seeks to ascertain the likelihood that one of a number of violent acts, such as robbery or assault, may occur towards an unidentified person within a broad societal context. We are not talking about assessment of stalking, or what may otherwise be referred to as targeted violence and the subsequent threat assessment. We are also not focusing on *Tarasoff* situations, in which clinicians assess for imminent violence of a client. Kropp, Hart, and Lyon (2002) point out some of these differences. Stalking is unique in that it has as a target for the violence a specific person. Stalking may include perceived, implied, or actual threats that may not be considered as violent in general risk assessment. Stalking may also persist over a long period of time whereas most general risk assessment outcomes are relatively short term from 1–5 years, though some extend to as many as 10 years. Further, the assessment of stalking does not have behind it the same breadth of empirical information from which more general violence assessment has benefited. Moreover, this book is specific to the assessment of violence in adults. While many risk factors are similar between adolescents and adults, both their assessment and content differ due to developmental differences. Other resources are available when assessing juveniles or young offenders for general violence (e.g., Borum & Verhaagen, 2006) or sexual violence (e.g., Barbaree & Marshall, 2008).

There is an interesting finding within the literature that nonviolent offending is a risk factor for sexual violence (Hanson & Thornton, 2000), spousal violence (Hilton et al., 2004), violence among offenders with mental disorders (Quinsey, Harris, Rice, & Cormier, 2006), and violence among violent criminals (Hollin & Palmer, 2003; Mills, Kroner, & Hemmati, 2003). It would appear, then, that individuals who commit nonviolent offenses are themselves at risk for committing a violent act at some point in the future. Research by Glenn Walters (2007) has supported the dimensional nature of the criminal lifestyle. Walters's research asked the question, Is there a type of person who is criminal or is criminal behavior better represented as gradations on a continuum? Walters's findings suggest that the latter is the case, with more entrenched offenders having more risk factors present. The presence of these risk factors can distinguish between those who will be violent and those who will not be violent once released from custody.

Despite the shared risk factors for different types of violence, there are also unique risk factors for each kind of violence. In the paragraphs to follow we outline the risk factors for violence among criminal recidivists, offenders with mental disorders (OMDs), sexual offenders, and those who commit intimate partner violence. In addition, we look at the specific role of psychopathy in the assessment of violence risk.

VIOLENT REOFFENDING IN THE CRIMINAL RECIDIVIST

Much study has gone into the specific risk factors that are related to violence. Many studies included both general recidivism and violence recidivism as outcomes. In most instances general recidivism has included violent reoffending. Therefore, violent recidivism is a subset of general recidivism. This frequently results in the same risk variables predicting both general and violent recidivism. As an example, the Level of Service Inventory—Ontario Version (Andrews, Bonta, & Wormith, 1995) also known as the Level of Service/Case Management Inventory (Andrews, Bonta, & Wormith, 2004) was used to predict both general and violent recidivism among correctional offenders released to the community (Girard & Wormith, 2004). All of the risk factors measured, which included criminal history, education/employment history, family and marital problems, leisure/recreation, companions, procriminal attitudes, and substance abuse were significantly correlated with any reconviction (Girard & Wormith, 2004). These same risk factors were also significantly correlated with violent reconviction and severity of the offense. Not surprisingly, criminal history was the most strongly related to each of these three outcomes. Practically speaking, most risk factors that predict general recidivism in correctional offenders also predict violence and severity of offending. Hollin and Palmer (2003) found that violent offenders within the British prison system had more criminal offenses, more antisocial companions, poorer educational background, and more alcohol and drug problems. It should not come as a surprise that offenders with more criminogenic needs (dynamic risk factors that can respond to intervention such as unemployment and substance abuse) and criminal history commit more offenses and are at greater risk for violence.

A study of primarily violent men serving sentences of 2 years or more in Canada showed that criminal history, education/employment deficits, financial problems, family and marital problems, antisocial companions, alcohol/drug problems, and emotional difficulties were all related to violent recidivism (Mills, Kroner, & Hemmati, 2003). These same variables, with the exception of emotional difficulties, predicted nonviolent recidivism in the same sample. An analysis of the HCR-20 and the VRAG items identified risk factors for violence in a similar sample (Mills, Kroner, & Hemmati, 2007). These included previous violence, young age at first violent incident, relationship instability, employment problems, early maladjustment, prior supervision failure, lack of insight, negative attitudes, impulsivity, unresponsiveness to treatment, plans lacking feasibility, exposure to destabilizers in the community, lack of personal support, noncompliance with remediation attempts, stress, elementary school maladjustment, separation from parents under the age of 16, failure on prior conditional release, and alcohol abuse.

Studies of violent offenders have shown that risk appraisal instruments that predict general recidivism also predict violent recidivism and conversely those that predict violent recidivism also predict general recidivism. Some of our own work has demonstrated that instruments that were developed to predict general recidivism such as the Level of Service Inventory—Revised and the Lifestyle Criminality Screening Form predicted both general and violent recidivism with equal accuracy (Kroner & Mills, 2001). Similar results were found with the HCR-20 and the VRAG, which were specifically developed to assess for violence likelihood. Our colleagues found similar results with a sample of predominantly violent correctional inmates (Glover, Nicholson, Hemmati, Bernfeld, & Quinsey, 2002).

Edward Zamble and Vern Quinsey (1997) studied men who had reoffended and were returned to custody to determine what they experienced in the community prior to committing their most recent offense. As part of this investigation they compared assaulters, robbers, and property offenders. Assaulters were much more likely to be employed than were robbers and property offenders. More assaulters identified interpersonal conflict as a problem than did robbers and property offenders. However, robbers and property offenders were more likely than assaulters to report substance abuse as a problem. Robbers were most likely to identify money or financial problems. This study was retrospective, so while not definitive it does indicate that the experiences of those who commit violent acts may be different depending upon the violent act that occurred. The same study showed that offenders who *do not* return to custody were more involved in family activities, more often had a prosocial hobby, spent less idle time listening to music and just "hanging around," and were much less likely to be socially isolated and less often reported being bored (Zamble & Quinsey, 1997). A summary of the more common static and potentially dynamic violence risk factors for the criminal recidivist are reported in Table 2.1.

Criminal activity in general puts individuals at risk for violence. A general antisocial orientation together with a criminal or antisocial milieu is a precursor for violence. This has been shown to be true for the correctional offender as well as among OMDs and patients within forensic psychiatric facilities (Quinsey, Harris, Rice, & Cormier, 2006). However, there are additional risk factors for violence among OMDs just as there are for specific types of violence such as sexual violence and spousal violence.

OFFENDERS WITH MENTAL DISORDERS

Mental illness is often believed to be the cause of crime and violence. However, research has shown that the link between mental illness and crime/violence is not as strong as one might think. One example is a study of seriously mentally ill individuals who had the role of their mental illness and substance abuse rated as either directly or indirectly contributing to the offense for which they were arrested (Junginger, Claypoole, Laygo, & Crisanti, 2006). In this study, 113 arrestees met the study's inclusion criteria of having a current serious mental illness defined as a DSM Axis I schizophrenia spectrum or major mood disorder and co-occurring substance use disorder. Subsequent ratings revealed that in only 4% of cases were the symptoms of the mental illness directly related to the offense for which they were arrested and in an additional 4% of cases the mental illness had an indirect effect on the offense. Substance abuse, however, played a much more significant role: in 19% of cases it was considered to have a direct effect on the offense and in an additional 7% of cases it was considered to have had an indirect effect on the offense.

The purpose of this section is to provide information on the relationship between OMDs and violence. Knowing about the relationship between mental illness and violence will provide a necessary context when communicating the risk for violence at an idiographic level and will provide guidance when making recommendations regarding the management of that risk. As a discipline, our understanding of this relationship is increasing, but this increase has not been uniform, and at times may appear contradictory. Some reasons for this include issues related to defining both mental illness and the outcome of violence. *Mental illness* has been used to refer to a heterogeneous group of psychiatric disorders, psychotic symptoms, schizophrenia only, major mental disorders, overnight stay in a psychiatric unit, or even referrals to a psychiatric unit. In some instances personality disorders (e.g., antisocial personality disorder, borderline personality disorder) have been

TABLE 2.1. Summary of Risk Factors among Criminal Recidivists

Static	Potentially dynamic
Childhood antisocial behavior	Employment/financial problems
Adolescent antisocial behavior	Current substance abuse
Age of first adult conviction	Family instability
Prior incarcerations	Criminal associates
Prior convictions for assaultive behavior	Antisocial attitudes/cognitions
Supervision failure	Mood problems/hostility
History of alcohol abuse	Resistance to intervention/supervision
Failure to complete high school	Unstructured leisure/criminal environment
Prior criminal associations	
Prior interpersonal difficulties	

considered mental disorders. Problems with the definition of violence are not unique to studies of OMDs but have included criminal charges, arrests, self-report, reports of others, multiple records, or threats. In addition to problems of definition, how mental health functioning has been measured also contributes to the varied mental illness—violence relationships. Types of measurement have included current diagnosis, past diagnosis, clinical records, structured diagnostic interviews, self-report, file ratings, and client ratings.

The type of sample being studied can also make a difference in the relationship between mental disorder and violence. Typically, three basic samples have been used to examine the violence–mental illness relationship: psychiatric patients, offenders, and epidemiological community-based studies (Arboleda-Flórez, 1998). Using only a psychotic patient sample to draw conclusions regarding a problem area, such as employment, crime, and homelessness, one may infer that mental illness is an explanatory factor for the difficulties that the individual is experiencing (Drain, Salzer, Culhane, & Hadley, 2002). Moreover, biases can be introduced when comparisons are made within groups or between groups. For example, the rate of violence for patients with schizophrenia is lower when compared to patients with other psychotic disorders or substance abuse. Similarly, the rate of violence for patients with schizophrenia is lower when compared with other individuals referred for psychiatric evaluations. However, when compared to the general population, those with schizophrenia tend to be at higher risk for violence (Walsh, Buchanan, & Fahy, 2002). So whether or not schizophrenia is a risk factor or a protective factor largely depends on the sample that is being studied. More will be said on this relationship a little later.

While most of the research on the seriously mentally ill is of a retrospective nature, the MacArthur study was a prospective study that should be considered a major advance in the field (Monahan et al., 2001). This study included more than 3,000 patients, 939 of whom were involved in a prospective study of violence risk. There were three different sites: Pittsburgh, Pennsylvania; Kansas City, Missouri; and Worcester, Massachusetts. The study considered 134 risk variables. *Violence* was defined as acts resulting in physical injury, assaultive acts with a weapon, or threats with a weapon. In addition, multiple sources were used to indicate violence. This prospective design has led to stronger conclusions regarding the role of mental illness in predicting violence. Within this study, serious mental illness was not related to later community violence. The best predictors in order of effect size included psychopathy (likely due to the antisocial history component; see later in this chapter), severity of prior adult arrests, frequency of prior adult arrests, antisocial personality disorder, drug or alcohol disorder, angry behavior, recent violent behavior, and arrest for a crime against a person. In fact, serious mental illness in the absence of substance abuse was negatively associated with violence. It is good to remember that while people with serious mental illness get arrested more often, the amount of societal violence attributable to serious mental illness is small. However, among the mentally ill there are a number of risk factors for violence worth noting.

A meta-analysis conducted by Bonta, Law, and Hanson (1998) examined the risk factors associated with the violence perpetrated by offenders with mental disorders. These researchers classified the various risk factors into demographic, criminal history, deviant lifestyle history, and clinical factors. Among the better demographic and criminal history predictors associated with violence were age, criminal history, nonviolent criminal history, history of violence, and institutional adjustment. Interestingly, whether or not the *index offense* (the offense for which the offender had been incarcerated) was violent was not related to later violence: what mattered most was the pattern of prior violent behavior. Among the deviant lifestyle history variables a lack of education, employment problems, and family problems were among the better predictors. Substance abuse was significant but the effect size was smaller. The clinical risk factor with the largest effect size was a diagnosis of antisocial personality disorder. This risk factor would share a lot of the similar features with a history of antisocial behavior. Prior hospitalizations was a smaller but significant risk factor, though interestingly days in hospital were negatively associated with violence. Intelligence and mood disorder were not related to future violence. However, a diagnosis of psychosis and being found not guilty by reason of insanity were negatively related to future violence. Finally, objective measures of risk were significantly superior to clinical judgment in the assessment for future violence. Many of these findings have been supported by research that has been conducted since the completion of this meta-analysis. The following paragraphs consider some of these risk factors in more detail.

The meta-analysis discussed was limited by the research that was available and surveyed and did not include many dynamic risk variables. Subsequent research has focused on identifying which potentially dynamic risk factors will predict the outcome of OMDs eloping from custody or reoffending. Quinsey, Coleman, Jones, and Altrows (1997) measured five problem areas (psychotic behaviors, skill deficits, inappropriate and procriminal social behaviors, mood problems, and social withdrawal) 6 months before the outcome and four proximal indicators (dynamic antisociality, psychiatric symptoms, poor compliance, and medication compliance/dysphoria) 1 month before the outcome. Of the combined nine areas studied, seven significantly differentiated between elopers/offenders and matched controls after controlling for static risk as measured by the VRAG. The seven variables were inappropriate and procriminal social behaviors, mood problems, social withdrawal, dynamic antisociality, psychiatric symptoms, poor compliance, and medication compliance/dysphoria. These same seven areas also differentiated the eloper/offender group at the time of the event as compared to the same individuals at a time prior to the event.

In a large, multiwave study, Quinsey, Jones, Book, and Barr (2006) developed a 29-item dynamic prediction scale to predict any incident (general risk) and violent incidents (violence risk). This scale was completed by the clients' caregiver and had General Risk and Violent Risk subscales. With a substantial sample ($n = 568$), Quinsey et al. conducted a truly prospective study. They assessed their clients (forensic mental health patients) monthly for an average of 33 months. During the follow-up period there were 256 incidents, which occurred both in the hospital and in the community. Patients with and without violent incidents were compared. Those with violent incidents had reportedly more current antisociality, more psychiatric symptoms, poorer medication compliance, poorer therapeutic alliance, and denied current problems. However, when within-comparisons were made looking at only those with violent incidents and comparing their performance in the months before the incident, inappropriate behaviors, mood problems, and therapeutic alliance tended to be the more significant risk factors (Quinsey, Book, & Skilling, 2004).

It is no surprise that substance abuse, which could also be considered a dynamic risk factor, has consistently been associated with violence among those with mental illness (Cuffel, Shumway, Choulijian, & Mac-Donald, 1994; Swartz et al., 1998; Teplin, Abrams, & McClelland, 1994). With violent offenders who had schizophrenia, substance abuse/dependence remained a significant predictor, even after controlling for psychopathy (Tengström, Grann, Långström, & Kullgren, 2000). In contrast, once age and psychopathy were accounted for, substance abuse did not add to the prediction of violence (Villeneuve & Quinsey, 1995). In studies that examined dual diagnoses, the likelihood of violence increased with the presence of substance abuse (Mullen, Burgess, Wallance, Palmer, & Ruschena, 2000). The rate of violence has been shown to go from 6.98% with a major mental illness to 22.02% with a dual diagnosis (Swanson, Holzer, Ganju, & Jono, 1990). This study also found that having more than one diagnosis and the presence of substance abuse resulted in more serious violent behavior and that the violence occurred at a higher frequency. In a large, multisite study of people with schizophrenia, co-occurring substance abuse/dependence was a predictor of minor violence (Swanson et al., 2006). In a large epidemiological study, once substance abuse was accounted for, mental illness symptomatology was not significant in the prediction of violence (Swartz & Lurigio, 2007). From these and other studies (Arsenault, Moffitt, Caspi, Taylor, & Silva, 2000; Brennan, Mednick, & Hidgins, 2000; Steadman et al., 1998) it appears that substance abuse is a main contributor, or at least has an interactive or additive effect, on the risk of violence. Polysubstance abusers are also at increased risk for violence (Cuffel et al., 1994).

From a developmental perspective it appears that boys with callous–unemotional traits and conduct disorder will be at increased likelihood to be persistently violent into adulthood. This group continues to have adult difficulty in identifying situations that have a possible negative outcome (Hodgins, 2007). Having a history of learning difficulties has also been found to be predictive of future violence among those with severe mental illness (Walsh et al., 2001); however, attention-deficit/hyperactivity disorder (ADHD) now appears not to have a direct role in persistent violence. As a group, those with ADHD are heterogeneous, with future violence being mediated by intelligence and psychosocial functioning (Mill et al., 2006). Early victimization has consistently been shown to be associated with future violence in the general population. Specifically, for those who have a mental disorder, victimization was predictive of violence in both the MacArthur and Duke Mental Health studies (Hiday, 2006).

Using data from the MacArthur study, Robins, Monahan, and Silver (2003) examined differences between men and women on violence and other aggressive acts. Surprisingly, no differences between the men and women occurred in violence over the 1-year follow-up. With regard to the targets of violence, family members were more likely to be a target of women than of men for both violence and other aggressive acts. Thus, violence committed by mentally ill women may not be as visible and not as readily detected by authorities. This may contribute to the underestimation of violent transactions committed by women with mental illness. Further support for an underestimation comes from the Swanson et al. (2006) study. Among those with schizophrenia, females contributed to more minor violence than did males. For serious violence there were no gender differences. With regard to predictors of violence, it appears that the predictors are similar for women and men, with past criminal history being the strongest predictor (Dean et al., 2002; Putkonen, Komulainen, Virkkunen, Eronen, & Lonnquist, 2003).

Of all the mental disorders, schizophrenia has garnered the most attention when examining crime and violence. For reasons mentioned above, the rates of mental illness and violence and the relationship between mental illness and violence have varied. While a number of studies suggest that having schizophrenia increases the likelihood of crime or violence (Brennan et al., 2000; Mullen et al., 2000; Wallace, Mullen, & Burgess, 2004), other studies suggest a null or negative relationship between schizophrenia and crime or violence (Feder, 1994; Harris, Rice, & Quinsey, 1993; Hodgins & Cote, 1993; Villeneuve & Quinsey, 1995; Quinsey et al., 2006). Even when a relationship between schizophrenia and violence is shown, often this relationship can be explained by substance use and/or antisocial personality disorder (Hiday, 2006). Overall, there is a weak positive relationship between schizophrenia and violence, but, as noted, one must be careful not to read causation into this relationship.

Affective disorders have traditionally been associated with aggression (Good, 1978); however, current research suggests that depression is not as powerful a risk factor in the prediction of violence as once thought. In the MacArthur study the presence of depression at the time of hospital admission had a near zero correlation with violence (–.003; Monahan et al., 2001, Table B1). Other studies also showed a negative relationship between violence and depression, suggesting that depression may inhibit the occurrence of violence (Beal, Kroner, & Weekes, 2003; McNeil, Eisner, & Binder, 2003).

As with other offenders, OMDs have considerable employment and housing difficulties. Despite this problem, two of the more utilized risk appraisal instruments (VRAG, HCR-20) do not substantially address the areas of employment and place of residence. Yet these areas, when measured, are consistently central to a person's overall success (Andrews & Bonta, 2010; Drake, Wallach, & McGovern, 2005). The relationship among employment, education, and mental illness, however, may not be straightforward. The literature suggests that over time symptoms impact educational achievement, which subsequently impacts employment (Draine et al., 2002). More specifically, recent research has shown mental illness not to be the main cause of being homeless. This conclusion comes from two lines of research. First, the literature shows that the adult homeless have higher rates of mental illness than homeless families. The range of 12–15% drops to 7–9% when children are included in the analyses (Culhane, Averyt, & Hadley, 1998). Second is the research on homeless shelters. Multivariate studies of shelter use suggest no effect of mental illness on shelter use (Bassuk et al., 1997; Shinn et al., 1998). This research points to social structures having importance for the OMD, but the relationship between a lack of social structure and mental illness may not be direct.

Mental Illness and Imminent Violence: *Tarasoff* Considerations

Understanding and accounting for serious mental illness in a violence risk assessment is important, but as the above review demonstrates it is only one aspect of the assessment process. There may be, however, situations in which serious mental illness assessed during a violence risk assessment may require a *Tarasoff* assessment. The presence of acute, command hallucinations articulated with vivid recall and specific detail of an intended target may change the nature of the risk assessment to include a *Tarasoff* assessment. A duty to protect under *Tarasoff* stems from the risk for serious harm being foreseeable. It needs to be clear that the concept of "foreseeability" is a legal term which Quattrocchi and Schopp (2005) state includes "the likelihood of harm, the magnitude of the possible harm, circumstances affecting risk and the cost of interventions to prevent harm" (p. 111) and more generally is defined as the potential for harm that can be reasonably anticipated. There are conflicting findings relating acute symptoms of mental illness with violence.

Foreseeability may not be the same as having delusions, perceived threat, or fantasies. Many studies have shown delusions and perceived threat to explain violence (Link, Andrews, & Cullen, 1992; Link, Monahan, Steuve, & Cullen, 1999; Swanson et al., 1990; Swanson, Borum, Swartz, & Monahan, 1996; Swanson, Estroff, Swartz, & Borum, 1997); however, these studies were of a retrospective nature and the McArthur data did not find delusions or perceived threat to be predictive of violence (Appelbaum, Robbins, & Monahan, 2000). In the *Doyle* decision (*Doyle v. United States*) the responsibility of mental health professionals using fantasies in assessing potential harm was addressed. The patient was hospitalized for his homicidal remarks. The army psychiatrist and health team concluded that the fantasies were used to shock people. Two days after discharge the patient killed a security guard (Doyle). The court concluded that the victim was not "foreseeable and identifiable," and the patient's fantasies were "not enough" to demonstrate a "high risk." In another case involving a client with fantasies, the court cites *Doyle* and states, "Such statements are commonly expressed to psychiatrists and merely pose but do not answer the difficult question of whether or not danger is actually present" (*White v. United States*, p. 1289).

The research on the role of fantasies varies, but some general conclusions are offered by Gellerman and Suddath (2005). The prevalence of violent fantasies is similar for both offenders and nonoffenders. Within criminal populations, most of the research is of a retrospective design, which greatly restricts any causation conclusions. Thus, given the above summary and given that fantasies may result from many motivations, their use in risk assessment is currently not warranted. Even their use in a *Tarasoff* assessment will need to meet a clear foreseeability standard. Whereas Gellerman and Suddath take a research-informed approach, Quinsey et al. (2006) make a rationale argument against overriding a risk assessment when a specific threat is present. They state, "It is tough to get data on imaginary events" (p. 200). In practice, a specific threat that meets the criteria of *Tarasoff* is quite rare. When it does occur, particularly in relation to mental illness, usually interventions and the passage of time will alleviate the threat.

Table 2.2 summarizes the more common risk factors for violence among OMDs. The brief summary below may assist in placing your client's mental health variables within a relevant violence–mental illness context.

1. The closer the active symptoms are in temporal proximity to the targeted outcome, the more powerful the symptom is as a predictor. Symptoms upon admission are better than symptoms at discharge (Gray et al., 2003; McNiel & Binder; 1995; McNiel et al., 2003).
2. Symptoms are better predictors of violence among civil samples than samples with a criminal conviction (Villeneuve & Quinsey, 1995).
3. Psychotic symptoms are more predictive of violence in a hospital and less predictive of violence in the community (Gray et al., 2003; McNeil & Binder, 1995). When looking at pre- and postdeinstitutional time frames, one study found no difference in the rates of violence between the institutional and deinstitutional time-frames (Mullen et al., 2000).
4. More violence occurs when living with others (Swanson et al., 2006;

TABLE 2.2. Summary of Risk Factors for Violence among OMDs

Static	Potentially dynamic
Young age	Antisocial orientation/attitudes
History of violent behavior convictions or otherwise	Noncompliance with supervision
History of nonviolent criminal behavior	Noncompliance with medication
Institutional adjustment problems	Mood disturbance/hostility
Poor education and employment history	Current alcohol/substance use
History of interpersonal/family problems	
History of alcohol/substance abuse	

Straznickas, McNeil, & Binder, 1993). The majority of violence by people who have mental illness occurs against family members.

5. The more risk factors related to criminal and violent behavior that are measured, the less mental health variables incrementally contribute to the prediction of violence (Steadman et al., 1998; Teplin et al., 1994).

SEXUAL VIOLENCE

Rates of sexual offending vary considerably depending on a number of factors and there is a general consensus that the actual recidivism rates are not known (Heilbrun, Nezu, Keeney, Chung, & Wasserman, 1998). Andrew Harris and Karl Hanson (2004) identified three factors that make determining actual recidivism rates a challenge. These include the definition, the follow-up period, and the diversity among sex offenders. Broader definitions such as using prostitutes or making threats would serve to increase rates of offending. Longer follow-up periods also serve to increase recidivism rates, though with each successive year the marginal rates tend to decline. Another important factor is the type of offender and offense. As an example, incest offenders have lower rates of recidivism when compared with child molesters who target unknown victims. Within the context of research, studies vary their definition of recidivism to include reconvictions, rearrests, or suspensions due to breaches of release conditions. Most important, as has already been said, recidivism almost always refers to officially detected behavior: it is a reasonable assumption that there is much undetected recidivism. An aggregate sample (10 samples combined) of just over 4,700 sex offenders confirmed that recidivism rates (defined as new charges and/or convictions) increased over time, varied with the age of the offender, increased with the presence of prior sexual convictions, and varied by type of victim (Harris & Hanson, 2004; see Table 2.3).

Notably, there is also a steady decline in recidivism rates among sexual offenders after the age of 40 (Hanson, 2006). This was found to be the case whether or not actuarial risk was controlled. The 5-year recidivism rate for offenders over the age of 60 years was only 2%, much lower than the 14.8% for offenders younger than 40 years of age. Because older and younger offenders may be grouped together within risk categories, this finding suggests that the Static-99 and other similar instruments may overestimate the recidivism rates of older offenders.

As with prediting other forms of violence, predicting sexual violence recidivism has changed from a focus on purely static and historical variables (Hanson, 1997; Hanson & Thornton, 2000) to assessments that include dynamic variables related to risk (Hanson, Harris, et al., 2007; Olver et al.,

TABLE 2.3. Sex Offender Recidivism Rates Over Time

Group	5 years	10 years	15 years
Whole sample	14.0% (12.9–15.1)	19.8% (18.5–21.5)	24.2% (22.2–25.8)
Rapists	14.1% (11.6–16.4)	20.6% (17.8–24.2)	24.1% (20.1–27.9)
Child molesters, extended incest	6.4% (4.1–7.9)	9.4% (5.6–12.4)	13.2% (7.7–18.3)
Child molesters, girl victims	9.2% (7.3–10.7)	13.1% (10.4–15.6)	16.3% (12.7–19.3)
Child molesters, boy victims	23.0% (19.4–26.6)	27.8% (23.8–32.2)	35.4% (29.3–40.7)

Note. Data from Harris and Hanson (2004). Parentheses contains 95% confidence intervals.

2007). This change was driven, in part, by the necessity of identifying points of intervention to reduce risk (Hanson & Harris, 2000) and by empirical findings from meta-analyses that identified dynamic variables as potent contributors to the prediction of sexual recidivism (Hanson & Bussiere, 1998; Hanson & Morton-Bourgon, 2005).

Hanson and Bussiere (1998) examined 87 research documents from various countries that examined sex offender recidivism in a total sample representing nearly 29,000 sexual offenders. This study reported on the relationship of variables both to sexual reoffense and to nonsexual violent recidivism. The average rate of sexual recidivism was 13.4% (18.9% for rapists and 12.7% for child molesters). The recidivism rate for nonsexual violence was 12.2% (22.1% for rapists and 9.9% for child molesters). A majority of studies defined *recidivism* as reconviction but some studies also considered arrests, self-reports, and parole violations. From their meta-analysis, Hanson and Bussiere identified a number of risk factors associated with sexual violence; those with stronger effect sizes included phallometric assessment with a preference for children, MMPI Masculinity–Femininity, severely disordered, any deviant sexual preference, prior sex offenses, failure to complete treatment, negative relationship with mother, any personality disorder, and stranger victim.

As can be seen from these meta-analytic results, a number of risk factors predict both sexual violence and nonsexual violence in sex offenders. Most notably are young age, antisocial personality (antisocial personality disorder and MMPI Psychopathic Deviate), prior nonsexual offenses, and being single. Being a rapist was positively correlated with nonsexual violence. A history of juvenile offending and prior violent behavior were also related to nonsexual violence. Variables that were not related to sexual reoffense included denial of the sex offense ($r = .02$), low motivation for treatment ($r = .01$), being sexually abused as a child ($r = -.01$), any substance abuse problem ($r = .03$), and alcohol abuse problem ($r = .00$).

In a later update and extension of earlier work, Hanson and Morton-Bourgon (2005) examined 115 published reports of sex offender recidivism from nine countries. In this meta-analytic review the authors coded the predictor variables into one of seven categories: sexual deviancy, antisocial orientation, sexual attitudes, intimacy deficits, adverse childhood environment, general psychological problems, and clinical presentation. The authors identified sexual deviancy and antisocial orientation as the major predictors, sexual attitudes and intimacy deficits as significant but relatively small predictors, and adverse childhood environment, general psychological problems, and clinical presentation as having "little to no relationship with sexual recidivism" (p. 1157). Importantly, they also identified a number of risk factors that they characterized as potentially misleading; that is, those risk factors that may appear to have an intuitive connection to recidivism but were not supported by the empirical findings. These include force or violence used in sex offending, neglect or abuse experienced during childhood, sexual abuse experienced during childhood, loneliness, low self-esteem, having a lack of victim empathy, denying the sexual crime, having a low motivation for treatment at intake, and a posttreatment evaluation of poor progress. Even those sophisticated in risk assessment could easily see how characterizations of an offender as denying all aspects of the offense, being poorly motivated, and making poor progress in treatment could easily override statistical information on the individual's likelihood to reoffend.

In a study sponsored by the U.S. Department of Justice, Knight and Thornton (2007) examined nine risk assessment instruments developed to predict sex offender sexual violence recidivism. Part of their study included a factor analysis of all of the individual items, similar in approach to that taken by Kroner, Mills, and Reddon (2005), to determine the structure underlying current sex offender appraisal instruments. The items formed five factors which they called Criminal Persistence, Sexual Persistence, Young and Single, Violent Stranger, and Male Victim Choice. Interestingly, only the factors of Sexual Persistence and Male Victim Choice approached a predictive accuracy rate similar to the risk appraisal instruments.

Dynamic Risk Factors

Measuring and including dynamic risk factors in the assessment of risk for sexual recidivism has received increased attention in recent years. Various methods have been employed to measure dynamic risk factors including those that rely upon psychometric self-report measures (Allan, Grace, Rutherford, & Hudson, 2007; Beech, 1998; Thornton, 2002) and those that rely upon assessor ratings (Hanson & Harris, 2001; Olver et al., 2007). The latter method of relying upon assessor ratings has shown more applied promise for the practitioner.

A study by Michael Allan and colleagues (2007) is typical of the self-report measure approach to assessing dynamic risk factors. A large test battery was administered to child molesters which covered the domains of sexual attitudes and beliefs, emotional functioning, and interpersonal functioning. Among the psychometric test battery were tests such as the Abel–Becker Cognitions Scale (Abel et al., 1989), the Hostility Towards Women Scale (Check, 1985), the Rape Myth Acceptance Scale (Burt, 1980), the Wilson Sexual Fantasy Questionnaire (Wilson, 1978), the Beck Depression Inventory (Beck, Steer, & Brown, 1997), the State–Trait Anxiety Inventory (Spielberger, 1983), the State–Trait Anger Expression Inventory (Spielberger, 1988), the Social Self-Esteem Inventory (Lawson, Marshall, & McGrath, 1979), the Assertion Inventory (Gambrill & Richey, 1975), the revised UCLA Loneliness Scale (Russell, Peplau, & Cutrona, 1980), the Fear of Intimacy Scale (Descutner & Thelen, 1991), the Adult Nowicki–Strickland Internal–External Locus of Control Scale (Nowicki & Duke, 1983), and the Marlowe–Crowne Social Desirability Scale (Crowne & Marlowe, 1960). Without going any further in the description of the study you can see quite readily why the application of the findings would be difficult indeed to translate into applied practice. A factor analysis of these scales was undertaken and four underlying factors were identified: sexual inadequacy, sexual interests, anger/hostility, and pro-offending attitudes. Each of these factors independently predicted sexual recidivism. In addition a composite "deviancy score" derived from the four factors also predicted sexual recidivism. These researchers then proceeded to determine if the "dynamic" information contained in the four factors could add to the Static-99 in the prediction of sexual reoffense. In fact, the sexual interests score, pro-offending attitudes score, and overall deviancy score all improved the prediction of recidivism over the Static-99 alone. There is growing evidence that the inclusion of construct measures related to the outcome of interest can improve the accuracy of purely historical information in the prediction of recidivism. The challenge is no longer so much in demonstrating the relevance of outcome-related constructs as in making the dynamic constructs easily measured and applied within a clinical context.

Moving from meta-analytic and empirical investigations to real-world applications associated with the measurement of risk factors is a challenge. To that end there have been two significant advances by researchers to develop risk assessment measures that include dynamic items that can be reliably measured and applied to the sexual violence risk assessment enterprise. Karl Hanson and Andrew Harris initiated the measurement of dynamic risk factors for sexual recidivism with the publication of their Sex Offender Need

Assessment Rating (SONAR; Hanson & Harris, 2001). Later revisions lead to the development of the Stable-2000 and the Acute-2000 and more recently the Stable-2007 and Acute-2007 (Hanson, Harris, et al., 2007), wherein these same researchers classified the dynamic variables into those that can change over a moderate period of time (Stable) and those that can change rather quickly (Acute). Dynamic *stable* variables include significant social influences, intimacy deficits (capacity for relationship stability, emotional identification with children, hostility toward women, general social rejection/loneliness, and lack of concern for others), general self-regulation (impulsive acts, poor cognitive problem-solving skills, negative emotionality/hostility), sexual self-regulation (sexual preoccupation, sex as coping, deviant sexual interests), and cooperation with supervision. The dynamic *acute* items include victim access, hostility, sexual preoccupation, and rejection of supervision when predicting sexual and violent recidivism. However, when predicting general recidivism three additional items are considered: emotional collapse, collapse of social supports, and substance abuse.

Hanson, Harris, et al. (2007) reported on the Dynamic Supervision Project that followed 978 sex offenders after they were released to the community. These offenders were assessed with both static (Static-99) and dynamic (Stable-2000 and Acute-2000) risk factors. The offenders were drawn from across Canada and two U.S. states and were followed for an average of 41 months postrelease. Among the outcomes of interest were sexual crimes (any sexual crime including noncontact and consenting such as prostitution) and any sexual recidivism (includes sexual crime recidivism as well as breaches for violations related to sexual offending). Sixteen items from the Stable-2000 were analyzed but the results supported the inclusion of only 13 items in the revised Stable-2007. Changes to the Acute-2000 resulted in four items related to the prediction of sexual and violent reoffending and seven items to the prediction of any reoffending within the Acute-2007 (see Table 2.4).

It is interesting to observe that none of the Stable variables were particularly strong performers in terms of prediction, but collectively in the Stable-2007 they improved accuracy, and when added to the Static-99 they improved overall accuracy even further. As noted previously, only four items of the Acute-2007 were associated with sexual recidivism (victim access, hostility, sexual preoccupations, and rejection of supervision). Together these variables added to both the Static-99 and the Stable-2007 in the prediction of recidivism. The Dynamic Supervision Project accomplished a significant step forward in the assessment and management of sexual violence. Several lessons were learned from this study.

Among these lessons are that not all of the variables previously thought to be associated with sexual recidivism were actually helpful in improving predictive accuracy. These include feelings of sexual entitlement, rape atti-

TABLE 2.4. Accuracy (AUC) of the Dynamic Supervision Project Predictors

Predictors	Sexual crimes	Any sexual recidivism
Static-99	.74	.69
Stable-2007	.67	.69
Acute-2007	.74	.65
Items of Stable-2007		
Significant social influences	.59	.60
Hostility toward women	.58	.59
General social rejection	.60	.61
Lack of concern for others	.58	.57
Sexual preoccupation	.58	.58
Sex as coping	.62	.60
Cooperation with supervision	.58	.62
Impulsive	.64	.64
Poor problem-solving skills	.60	.63
Negative emotionality	.55	.56
Capacity for relationship stability	.62	.62
Emotional identification with children	.52	.55
Deviant sexual preferences	.58	.58

Note. Data from Hanson, Harris, et al. (2007).

tudes, and child molester attitudes. Given the significance of these variables in other research, it is possible that the lack of association with sexual recidivism was due to difficulties in identifying and coding the variables in an actual clinical setting. This was somewhat underscored by the observation that the more conscientious parole/probation supervisors produced much more accurate results. It is possible that the measurement of the construct and not the actual construct itself is what resulted in these findings. For example, it is one thing to say that attitudes are related to sexual recidivism and quite another to measure those attitudes accurately within the applied context of supervision and then demonstrate that relationship. Further, Hanson, Harris, et al. (2007) concluded that although the dynamic items added to the predictive accuracy of the Static-99, there was little evidence that change in these items over time was related to recidivism. Therefore, although dynamic variables have been identified, relating changes in those variables to recidivism remains elusive. This would suggest that it is likely the construct represented by the dynamic variable (e.g., poor problem solving) as opposed to relatively little change in the construct that is adding to the predictive accuracy. Other risk factors for sexual violence that have increased the predictive accuracy of risk assessment instruments such as the Static-99 include a history of foster care, a history of substance abuse, a history of employment problems and/or instability, and a history of school maladjustment (Craig, Beech, & Browne, 2006). In addition to dynamic variables adding to static actuarial risk estimates, a notable interaction between risk factors has been replicated and found to improve prediction.

An interaction effect between psychopathic traits and sexual deviance in the prediction of sexual reoffense over the course of 10 years as been confirmed (Rice & Harris, 1997). Deviant psychopaths, those with a deviant phallometric result and a PCL-R score of 25 or greater, reoffended at a much higher rate than other sexual offenders. This interaction was confirmed in later works (Harris et al., 2003; Olver & Wong, 2006). Unfortunately, these studies used the PCL-R *total score* in the interaction term and did not report if the interaction was due to the total PCL-R score, Factor 1 (personality), or Factor 2 (lifestyle). This would have been an important distinction given the poor performance of Factor 1 in predicting sexual recidivism (Knight & Thornton, 2007). Table 2.5 provides a summary of the central risk factors for sexual violence.

SPOUSAL VIOLENCE

As with sexual violence and the violence of OMDs, the most consistently predictive risk factors for spousal violence are quite similar to those for

TABLE 2.5. Summary of Risk Factors for Sexual Violence

Static	Potentially Dynamic
Male victim	Sexual preoccupation
Prior sexual offenses	Lonely/single
Current or prior nonsexual offenses	Behaviorally impulsive
Unrelated or stranger victim	Emotional dysregulation/hostility/anger
Young age	Emotional identification with children
Personality disorder	Antisocial orientation/peers
Sexual deviance	Intimacy deficits/relationship instability
	Access to victims
	Uncooperative/noncompliant

violence in general with the addition of some unique risk factors that are specific to this type of violence. Also of note is that for spousal abuse there are fewer predictive studies than are available in the prediction of general violence and sexual violence. With this all said, there are important risk factors that are quite relevant and predictive of future spousal assault.

An example of the risk factors for general violence relevant to spouse assaulters were those identified in a large sample of male spouse assaulters who were attending community-based treatment programs (Hanson & Wallace Capretta, 2004). In other words, risk factors that predicted recidivism among general criminal populations also predicted future violence in a sample of spouse assaulters. These included such risk factors as younger age, prior arrests for assault, any prior convictions, poor performance at work or school, poor financial situations/management, criminal peers, and attitudes supportive of abuse. Unfortunately, the most limiting aspect of the study is that the criminal record check did not permit the identification of spouse assault and was limited to violence in general. Nonetheless, this evidence indicates that violence risk factors among spouse assaulters are very similar to violence risk factors in general.

Hilton, Harris, and Rice (2001) compared spouse assaulters with other offenders in a sample of offenders referred for mental health assessment in a maximum security psychiatric facility. Compared to other violent offenders, spouse assaulters were generally a lower risk group with a general violence recidivism rate of 24% compared with 44% for the comparison group over a 6- to 7-year time period. The VRAG risk appraisal instrument correlated with violence outcome as well with spouse assaulters as it did with the comparison group of offenders. It is important to note that the outcome here was general violence and not specifically spousal violence. Spouse assaulters had fewer psychopathic traits, tended to be older, tended to commit fewer crimes in general, fewer suffered from personality disorder, and had fewer failures during conditional release periods. It would appear then that many of the same risk factors predict general violence in violent offender and spouse assaulter populations but those risk factors may present to varying degree or with varying quantity among spouse assaulters. As an example, psychopathic traits predict general violence in mentally disorder and correctional populations, as it does among spouse assaulters; however, the average score on the PCL-R among spouse assaulters was considerably lower than other violent populations (see Hilton, Harris, Rice, Houghton, & Eke, 2008).

Reviews of the literature have identified specific risk factors such as having a lower socioeconomic status, a history of marital conflict, the existence of verbal and psychological abuse, having a more severe incident of spousal assault, and having a prior arrest for domestic violence. In addition to these specific risk factors, other risk factors that are common to other forms of violence include being younger, being at risk for general criminal behavior, substance abuse, and psychopathy (Hilton & Harris, 2005). It should come as no surprise that young age, criminal orientation, substance abuse, and psychopathy would be risk factors. All these can be reasonably associated with poor social and problem-solving skills, impulsivity, and general violence proclivity. In addition to psychopathy, the VRAG risk appraisal instrument has also been shown to be related to spouse abuse in equal terms with instruments such as the SARA, DA, and DVSI that were specifically designed for predicting spouse abuse (Hilton, Harris, et al., 2008).

In a study of spouse abusers Arlene Weisz and colleagues (Weisz, Tolman, & Saunders, 2000) examined a number of variables identified in the literature as potential risk factors for spouse abuse. They specifically examined serious violence within a brief time frame. In addition to victim and perpetrator characteristics researchers asked victims to rate on a scale of 0 (low) to 10 (high) the likelihood the perpetrator would become violent with them within the next year. Four months later in a follow-up interview victims were asked to report any incidence of serious violence. Correlated with serious spouse abuse were acts of violence or forced sex in the 6 months prior to the incident that brought the perpetrator to court (index offense). Also associated with this serious outcome was the presence of a protection order, whether the victim was treated for injuries because of the index offense, jealousy, threats, and attempts to control the victim. The risk factor with the second strongest relationship with outcome was additional violent incidents between the index offense and the court date, and the risk factor most strongly related to serious abuse was the victim's own prediction of the perpetrator's likelihood of becoming violent in a dispute with her within the next year ($r = .49$). Other research supports this finding that the victim's perception of risk of domestic violence may also be an important risk factor. For example, some have suggested that women who identify as high risk for spousal violence take precautions, whereas women who express uncertainty about their safety do not and are therefore more likely to experience reabuse (Heckert & Gondolf, 2004). Adding the victim's perception of risk also improved the predictive accuracy over perpetrator and victim characteristics alone.

Perpetrator personality may also predict spousal violence. The presence of a personality disorder is consistent with the findings of a birth cohort study reported by Terrie Moffitt and colleagues (Moffitt, Krueger, Caspi, & Fagan, 2000). At the age of 18, participants in the study were administered a measure of personality. When these participants reached the age of 21, they were interviewed again as part of the ongoing study methodology. The participants answered a questionnaire that pertained to criminal behavior they may have perpetrated over the past year. Factor analysis lent support to distinguishing between general crime and spouse abuse rather than treating the behaviors as uniform antisocial behaviors, but there remained a significant relationship between these two types of antisocial behavior. Negative Emotionality was consistently related to both crime in general and spouse abuse for both men and women with relatively equal coefficients. Constraint (self-control) was negatively correlated with both crime and spouse abuse though significantly more so for crime. In a separate analysis Constraint did not improve over Negative Emotionality in the prediction of spouse abuse but did improve the prediction of crime in general. The pattern held true for violent crime and violent spouse abuse. Those individuals who had higher Negative Emotionality and lower Constraint reported more violence both inside and outside the intimate relationship. These authors suggested that perpetrators of spouse abuse are more deliberate than impulsive as Constraint was not as strongly related to spouse abuse.

In addition to spousal assault in general, spousal homicide has received considerable attention. It should be noted that this latter outcome is very nearly impossible to predict with accuracy because of the very low base rate (i.e., spousal homicide is so statistically rare that accurate prediction is highly improbably if not impossible). A review of 22 empirical studies that examined the risk factors associated with spousal homicide indicated nine major risk factors (Aldridge & Browne, 2003). Individuals who witness family violence or who were themselves victims of family violence are at increased risk for spousal homicide. Women who were involved in common-law as opposed to marital relationships and women who were more than 10 years younger than their husbands were identified as being at greater risk. Drug and alcohol abuse by the male partner was identified as a significant risk factor, as was sexual jealousy. Separation or the threat of separation was also identified as a risk factor—most homicides occurred within the first year of separation. Men who stalked their spouses were also more likely to be fatally violent. The presence of a personality disorder in the perpetrator was also related to increased severity and frequency of violence. Finally, specific personality disorders were identified such as those with borderline or overcontrolled features. Risk factors associated with spousal homicide also inform on the risk factors associated with nonlethal spouse abuse as the majority of men who eventually kill their spouse have abused their spouse in the past (Moracco, Runyan, & Butts, 1998).

Risk factors identified in cases of criminal harassment/stalking are also closely aligned with risk factors in general. In a study of harassment and stalking cases in New York City, violence, defined as unwanted physical contact or confrontation with a weapon, was reported in 34% of cases (Rosenfeld & Harmon, 2002). The risk factors that distinguished the violent group from the nonviolent group included younger age, lower education, nonwhite, having a prior intimate relationship, prior threats, psychotic disorder diagnosed (less likely), having substance abuse diagnosis, and lower intellectual functioning.

A number of risk appraisal instruments have been developed to assess for the risk of spousal assault; however, relative to other types of outcome studies with general violence and sexual violence, the number of studies that report a risk appraisal instrument with a spouse assault outcome are fewer. For example, a meta-analysis of risk appraisal instruments that were used to predict spouse abuse identified only five studies that used or imputed the Spousal Assault Risk Assessment (Hanson, Helmus, & Bourgon, 2007). Curiously, assessment instruments like the VRAG and PCL-R were equal to or greater in predictive accuracy than instruments developed for the specific purpose of predicting spouse abuse. However, it needs to be noted that with such small numbers and the retrospective nature of the research, a definitive understanding of the predictive accuracy of these instruments has yet to be attained.

Among the spousal risk appraisal instruments is the Domestic Violence Supplementary Report (DVSR; Ontario Ministry of the Solicitor General, 2000), a 20-item instrument where the items are scored dichotomously. The instrument was developed primarily to assist frontline police officers to determine the number of risk factors present when responding to a domestic assault complaint. The DVSR items include substance abuse, compliance with court orders, mental illness, stalking of the victim, weapons, and patterns of jealousy. Another instrument, the Danger Assessment, developed by Campbell (1986, 1995), is a 15-item structured clinical assessment that was initially designed to assess the risk for serious harm or homicide of women in domestic violence circumstances. The Danger Assessment was one of the first instruments to show predictive validity in a short-term (3-month) follow-up of domestic violence (Goodman, Dutton, & Bennett, 2000).

The Spousal Assault Risk Assessment (SARA; Kropp, Hart, Webster, & Eaves, 1999) is a 20-item structured professional judgment instrument used to assess an individual's propensity for future spousal assault. The SARA is divided into two parts: Part 1 comprises risk factors more strongly associated with violence generally, whereas Part 2 comprises risk factors more strongly associated with spousal abuse specifically. Part 1 has been shown to be robustly associated with other measures of general and violent recidivism, whereas Part 2 does not share the same relationship (Kropp & Hart, 2000). A study conducted by Martin Grann and Ingela Wedin (2002) in Sweden showed that prior violations of conditional release, personality disorder with anger impulsivity and behavioral instability, and extreme minimization of assault history featured prominently as risk factors in their study of high-risk spouse abusers. Oddly, the risk factor of severity and/or sexual assault was inversely related to later recidivism.

The Ontario Domestic Assault Risk Assessment (ODARA; Hilton et al., 2004) is a more recently developed actuarial risk assessment instrument that incorporates probability estimates that set it apart from other structured instruments that do not assign probabilities to resulting scores. The ODARA's development and validity will be described in more detail in Chapter 3. At this point it should be noted that 35 perpetrator/victim characteristics were considered, 28 of which were significantly related to spousal assault; however, for practical purposes only the 13 strongest predictors were included in the final instrument. This finding underscores two issues that are related to risk assessment in general: the identification of specific risk factors and why instruments may differ in the assessment of risk. First, there were many more risk factors identified than could reasonably be considered in an assessment instrument. The final selection of these risk factors rests on the statistical procedure used and the specific nature of the sample. The same statistical procedure on a different sample may have yielded a slightly different set of risk factors. Among the risk factors identified that had a significant relationship with spouse assault that *did not* become a part of the ODARA are victim's age (negative relationship), victim being unemployed, perpetrator being unemployed, perpetrator being charged, duration of the relationship (negative relationship), number of prior criminal charges, and perpetrator's age (negative relationship). The reason for this development is the presence of multicollinearity among risk factors. More will be said about multicollinearity in the next chapter.

The successful treatment of spouse abusers appears to be elusive. Two recent reviews of risk factors for spousal violence concluded that there is no compelling evidence from the published literature that treatment programs are effective in reducing this type of violence (Catteneo & Goodman, 2005; Hilton & Harris, 2005). Some studies suggest success. For example, one study found that spousal abusers who completed a 14-session treatment program reoffended at a lower rate that those who failed to complete the program (Hendricks, Werner, Shipway & Turinetti, 2006); however, those who failed to complete the program included those who reoffended during the program as well as those refusing to enter the program. It is important to note that those offenders who fail treatment programs in general are typically higher risk offenders so there is a self-selection phenomenon at work to create this difference. Table 2.6 provides a summary of the more common risk factors for intimate partner violence.

PSYCHOPATHIC TRAITS

Theoretically, psychopathy is a personality disorder (not currently recognized in the DSM system of classification) reflected by a pattern of interpersonal, affective, and behavioral symptoms (Hare, 1996, 2003; Hart, Hare,

TABLE 2.6. Summary of Risk Factors for Spousal Violence

Static	Potentially dynamic
Prior domestic offense	Substance abuse
Current or prior non domestic offenses	Behaviorally impulsive
Prior incarceration	Emotional dysregulation/hostility/anger/jealousy
General violence toward others	Violation of noncontact orders/uncooperative/ noncompliant
Threats of serious harm toward victim	Relationship instability
Forced sex with spouse	Stalking spouse
Personality disorder	Perpetrator being unemployed
Victim's own prediction	
Confinement or control of victim	

& Harpur, 1992). Interpersonally, the prototypic psychopath is grandiose, egocentric, manipulative, dominant, forceful, and cold-hearted. Affectively, the psychopath is shallow with an inability to form enduring close relationships, demonstrates a significant lack of empathy, and is marked by an absence of anxiety, guilt, or remorse. Behaviorally, the psychopath is impulsive, sensation seeking, antisocial/criminal, and fails to fulfill social responsibilities. These descriptions are consistent with Cleckley's (1976) conceptualization of a prototypical psychopath. Within correctional populations, offenders with psychopathic traits tend to be arrested at an early age, commit more offenses and more violent offenses, spend more time incarcerated, experience more release failures, and exhibit institutional maladjustment (Wong, 1984). An important feature that has traditionally placed psychopathy within violence risk assessment is the consistent relationship between psychopathic traits and violence in general and instrumental violence in particular (Gacono, 2000; Hare & McPherson, 1984; Kosson, Steuerwald, Forth, & Kirkhart, 1997; Serin, 1991; Serin & Amos, 1995). Self-reports among those high on psychopathic traits have indicated that they view themselves as socially dominant and prone to respond aggressively (Morrison & Gilbert, 2001).

Theories on the etiology of psychopathy vary. Research conducted by Moffitt (1993) into persistent antisocial behavior over the life course suggests that it may be the result of some kind of neuropsychological or brain disorder occurring very early in life (i.e., prenatal, perinatal, and/or postnatal difficulties). These organic dysfunctions are thought to influence the development of antisocial behavior by undermining the development of social skills and emotional regulation. Another theory suggests that psychopathy is genetically determined and is an evolutionary adaptive strategy defined as a "genetically organized pattern for allocation of time, energy, and other resources to survival, growth, and reproduction during different periods of an organism's life" (Quinsey, Skilling, Lalumiere, & Craig, 2004, p. 101). Support for this latter theory comes from studies that have suggested psychopathy can be represented as a taxon (Harris, Rice, & Quinsey, 1994; Skilling, Harris, Rice, & Quinsey, 2002). Using the PCL-R (Hare, 1991, 2003) and the DSM-IV diagnostic criteria for antisocial personality disorder (American Psychiatric Association, 1994), Harris, Rice, and Quinsey (2002) concluded that there is a discrete class of men who exhibit a lifelong pattern of antisocial behavior. Similar analyses have been undertaken with boys with similar results. Skilling, Quinsey, and Craig (2001) applied taxometric analyses to several measures of antisocial behavior. The results suggested that there is a small but discrete class of boys who engage in serious antisocial behavior. We would also note that other researchers have failed to detect a taxon despite rigorous analysis (Edens, Marcus, Lilienfeld, & Poythress, 2006). Additional support for the theory of psychopathy as not originating from an organic abnormality comes from studies that examined the relationship of proxies for neuropsychological abnormalities and antisocial personality disorder (Coid, 1993), examinations of obstetrical complications in men who persistently acted out (Schulsinger, 1972), and comparisons of obstetrical complications and fluctuating asymmetry (a measure thought to be associated with underlying developmental difficulties) between psychopathic violent offenders with nonpsychopathic offenders (Lalumiere, Harris, & Rice, 2001). Regardless, a clear etiology for psychopathic traits has not been determined.

As noted above, psychopathic traits have been shown to be related to violence and intrinsic to psychopathy is a possible explanation for the violence: this is important to remember as we consider the backdrop to the rise of psychopathy as a construct important to forensic samples in the prediction of violence. During the 1970s and 1980s, following the conclusion that clinical judgment was ineffective in predicting violence, a growing need emerged for some measure that could reliably do so. Robert Hare had been studying and publishing research on the neurophysiology of psychopaths since the 1960s. In order to distinguish between psychopathic individuals and nonpsychopathic individuals he developed a 12-item checklist based on Cleckley's (1959) description of a prototypic psychopath (Hare, 1965, 1968). This checklist of "global ratings of psychopathy (on a 7-point scale), using Cleckley's (1976) conception of psychopathy" (p. 238) continued in his work into the 1970s (Hare, 1978). Hare published the first version of the Psychopathy Checklist (PCL) as a 22-item research scale in 1980 that was purportedly represented by five factors (Hare, 1980). The 22-item scale became the primary measure of psychopathy through the 1980s (Hare, 1982, 1984) and was quickly shown to be associated with violence in offender populations (Hare & McPherson, 1984), and later among mentally disordered populations (Harris et al., 1991). By the early 1990s, the demand for violence risk assessment was ever increasing, and there was no other measure that could match the empirical and theoretical force of psychopathy as a measure to aid in the prediction of violent behavior. Hence, psychopathy and the PCL were becoming synonymous and essential ingredients to the prediction of violence. Although other risk assessment measures became available, such as the Level of Supervision Inventory (LSI; Andrews, 1982; Andrews & Robinson, 1984), predecessor to the LSI—Revised (Andrews & Bonta, 1995), these latter instruments were identified with general recidivism and not violent recidivism in particular.

By 1990 Hare and colleagues published the revised Psychopathy Checklist (PCL-R) in *Psychological Assessment*. The 22-item scale had been reduced to a 20-item scale said to comprise two factors, "a selfish, callous, and remorseless use of others (Factor 1) and a chronically unstable, antisocial, and socially deviant lifestyle (Factor 2)" (p. 341). A screening version of the PCL-R was later developed (PCL: SV; Hart, Hare, & Forth, 1994; Hart, Cox, & Hare, 1995), as was a youth version (Forth, Kosson, & Hare, 2003). As the construct of psychopathy grew to prominence within correctional and forensic settings, in large part due to the use of the PCL-R, there was also a veritable explosion of research examining the validity of psychopathic traits in multiple populations, across offender types such as sex offenders and spouse abusers (Hilton et al., 2001), across culture and gender, and across varied outcome criteria. Another important development was the inclusion of psychopathy, specifically the PCL-R score, into two violence risk measures, the VRAG and the HCR-20. At this point if a clinician wanted to assess the likelihood for violence using two of the more prominent risk assessment measures, he or she would be required to score the PCL-R.

Out of the plethora of research on the PCL-R, questions began to arise about its underlying assumptions. For example, comparisons between the PCL-R and the LSI-R in terms of the relative predictive accuracy to predict general and violent offenses within criminal justice settings found that the LSI-R was a better predictor of general recidivism and modestly better than the PCL-R in predicting violent recidivism (Gendreau, Goggin, & Smith, 2002). In spite of tendencies for many to use the PCL-R as a violence risk predictor, Hemphill and Hare (2004) noted that the PCL-R does not assess risk, rather it "provides unique information that might help clinicians to understand better the offenders and patients with whom they work" (p. 207). Furthermore, the PCL-R manual specifically states that the instrument "provides a reliable and valid assessment of an important clinical construct—psychopathy. Strictly speaking, that is all that it does" (Hare, 2003, p. 15).

Meta-analyses have played a significant role in determining the relationship between psychopathic traits and antisocial behavior. To date at least 10 such analyses have been published.[1] These analyses examined the relationship of psychopathic traits as measured by the PCL instruments in both adults and adolescents, both males and females, and considering a variety of outcomes such as general, violent, and sexual recidivism. In six of these meta-analyses comparisons were available for the two factors in their relation with outcome and in each study the antisocial behavior factor (Factor 2), when reported, had a greater absolute relationship with outcome than did the personality/affective factor (Factor 1). In most cases the differences were considerable. For example, one of these meta-analyses found that Factor 2 was a significantly better predictor than Factor 1 in studies with male or adult participants, or with outcomes as varied as institutional adjustment, general recidivism, and violent recidivism (Walters, 2003b).

One of the more recent meta-analyses (Leistico et al., 2008) examined the relationship between the psychopathy checklists and outcome while considering a number of possible moderating factors. These moderating variables included age, country, race, gender, length of follow-up, institutional setting, information used to assess the PCL, and type of methodology. *Moderating variables* are those variables that may explain in part the relationship of the predictor variable with the outcome variable. The findings showed no difference in the effect size (the strength of the relationship of the PCL instruments with outcome) between the outcomes of institutional infractions and recidivism, between violent and nonviolent offenses, and across age groups.

In addition to age and type of outcome, the Leistico et al. (2008) study found that effect sizes for PCL Total and Factor 2 scores were smaller for samples in the United States than for samples from other places in the world. Similarly, effect sizes were smaller for non-Caucasian groups than for Caucasian participants. Effect sizes for Factor 2 scores were larger for participants from psychiatric hospitals than for offenders and they were larger for longer periods of follow-up than for shorter periods. The findings also showed that PCL Total and Factor 1 scores were larger in samples that included more female participants.

Glenn Walters and colleagues (Walters, Knigh, Grann, & Dahle, 2008) recently compared the incremental predictive validity of the PCL-R and the PCL: SV across six diverse samples that included civil psychiat-

---

[1]Edens and Campbell (2007); Edens, Campbell, and Weir (2007); Gendreau, Goggin, and Smith (2002); Gendreau, Little, and Goggin (1996); Guy, Edens, Anthony, and Douglas (2005); Hemphill, Hare, and Wong (1998); Leistico, Salekin, DeCoster, and Rogers (2008); Salekin, Rogers, and Sewell (1996); and Walters, (2003a, 2003b).

ric patients, prison inmates, sex offenders, and violent offenders. These researchers considered the relative contribution of the four facets of psychopathy in the prediction of violent and criminal behavior. Hare's revised manual (2003) proposed that the initial 2 factors could be further broken down into 4 facets (Affective, Interpersonal, Lifestyle, and Antisocial History). In general they found that when Facet 4 (Antisocial History) was entered into a predictive equation the remaining three facets failed to improve predictive validity. That is to say, that once antisocial history is considered, the remaining three facets of psychopathy (Lifestyle, Affective, Interpersonal) do not further explain criminal and violent behavior. Further analysis of Facet 4 revealed that it could be divided into a criminal component and a general acting-out component. The criminal component was more robustly linked to violence and recidivism, which led the authors to conclude that the facet was circular such that past criminal behavior was predicting future criminal behavior.

In addition to predictive differences observed between core personality characteristics (Factor 1) and antisocial/criminal behavior (Factor 2), research has suggested a three-factor model is a better representation of psychopathy (Cooke & Michie, 2001; Cooke, Michie, & Skeem, 2007). The three factors have been described by Cooke and Michie as Arrogant and Deceitful Interpersonal Style, Deficient Affective Experience, and Impulsive and Irresponsible Behavioral Style. Noticeably absent were the items that measure criminal behavior. From the discussion above regarding the predictive validity of Factor 2 that contains the historical items related to criminal behavior, it will quickly become apparent that by removing past criminal history from the measure of psychopathy it will reduce its association with future criminal and violent behavior. Among their conclusions, Cooke and Michie (2001) indicated that this was necessary because "conflating traits and behavior in the measurement of psychopathy means that it is impossible to infer that personality pathology drives antisocial behavior" (p. 185). A further interesting observation by these authors was that "the majority of the items that they [Harris et al., 1994] used to define the taxon have been dropped from the three-factor model. This suggests that the taxon, if is exists, is not psychopathy but may represent the life-course persistent offender taxon described by Moffitt (1993)" (p. 185).

The three-factor model of psychopathy was compared directly with the original two-factor solution and a subsequent two-factor, four-facet hierarchical model of the PCL-R (Hare, 2003), where Facets 1 (Interpersonal items) and 2 (Affective items) comprise Factor 1, and Facets 3 (Lifestyle items) and 4 (Antisocial items) comprise Factor 2 (Cooke et al., 2007). These authors found the three-factor solution generated a better fit (a better model) than either the original two-factor or subsequent two-factor, four-facet models.

They subsequently challenged the idea that criminal behavior was central to the construct of psychopathy. Citing their empirical findings they concluded "there is no compelling empirical evidence to support the conclusion that antisocial behavior is a central feature of psychopathy" (p. 248). Cooke et al. further indicated that Cleckley (1976) did not consider criminal behavior as central to psychopathy but rather as a possible outcome.

Jennifer Skeem and David Cooke (2010) directly challenge the notion that criminal behavior is central to psychopathy. Their contention is that psychopathy and the PCL-R may have become synonymous, wherein the measure and the construct are equated. They suggest that this perception has influenced the development of the understanding of psychopathy. Because criminal history is so prominent within the PCL-R scoring, they suggest that "without a history of violent or criminal behavior, even an individual with pronounced interpersonal and affective traits of psychopathy is unlikely to surpass the PCL-R's threshold score for diagnosing 'psychopathy'" (p. 434). They further observe that criminal behavior is associated with more than one type of pathology. Their full arguments will not be recapitulated here, but they make a compelling challenge to the existing conceptualization of psychopathy. No doubt this will serve to direct future research and quite possibly contribute to an evolution of our understanding of the construct.

Another development of late in the literature has been a change in the use of psychopathic traits within structured risk assessment instruments. For example, in a recent revision of their book on violent offenders, Quinsey et al. (2006) have provided an alternate measure to the PCL-R in the scoring of the VRAG and SORAG. The Childhood and Adolescent Taxon Scale (CATS; Quinsey, Harris, et al., 2006) measures the onset of serious antisocial behavior during childhood and adolescence, that is, the early onset of antisocial behavior. The CATS comprises nine items that are easily scored from an interview, with the resulting total providing a weighted score for inclusion in the VRAG in place of the PCL-R. The probability estimates of the VRAG remain the same so the substitution is seamless. Likewise, a revised version of the HCR-20 (HCR—Version 3), which is currently in field testing, will not require the scoring of the PCL-R (Kevin Douglas, personal communication, February 18, 2009). The replacement item will be structured to measure serious personality disorder which may include but is not limited to the use of the PCL-R.

From a research perspective, psychopathic traits are important risk factors for violence. However, there is growing evidence to suggest that it is the criminal history component that is responsible for most of the predictive validity. While others may differ, it seems to us that if the construct of psychopathy is composed of two factors and only one of those factors, the antisocial behavioral/criminal history component, is consistently related to violent outcome, then it is not psychopathic personality per se that is consistently related to violent outcome but rather the presence of a criminal history commonly shared by many offenders that is most instrumental in predicting future violent or criminal behavior.

Apart from including PCL-R scores within violence risk measures, we have been challenged clinically to find an effective way to integrate and explain subthreshold diagnostic scores within the context of a risk assessment. That is to say, if an offender's score is between 20 and 29 on the PCL-R (which corresponds to the middle range of scores), what does that information convey about the offender other than his score being similar to the majority of offenders within criminal justice settings? He is not "a psychopath" but frequently is described in reports (not ours) as scoring in the "moderate range of the PCL-R" or alternatively "his score relating to psychopathy was found to be at the 50th percentile." We have a concern that statements such as these lead the reader to understand the person to be "almost a psychopath" when in fact among many criminal samples the person is quite average. Support for this concern was found in work by Edens, Guy, and Fernandez (2003) who found that simply reporting some prototypic psychopathic personality characteristics was sufficient to increase the likelihood of recommending the death penalty among laypersons.

In our own sample (JFM and DGK) of nearly 1,500 mixed violent and sex offenders referred for a risk assessment who were serving sentences of 2 years or greater, the incidence of psychopathy (a score of 30 or greater on the PCL-R) was only 12%. Approximately 50% had scores below 20, with a remaining 38% having scores between 20 and 29. In this instance, half of the offenders were clearly not psychopathic. For the 38% who were clearly criminal but had some psychopathic traits, what does a score on the PCL-R mean? If the individual cannot be identified as a psychopath and only as "antisocial" then one runs the risk of introducing all of the potentially pejorative aspects of psychopathy without a definitive diagnosis. This was brought home to one of us (JFM) when a clerical assistant of a parole board expressed concerns regarding the assessment of a case because the offender being assessed was "almost a psychopath" (the offender had a PCL-R score in the high 20s). The availability of a score and knowledge of a cut-point for "psychopath" was clearly being utilized within the decision process by one unqualified to do so.

To date, the primary theories of psychopathy's etiology rely upon a biological/genetic explanation. Laboratory studies that serve as proxy research to support underlying biological/brain differences between psychopathic and nonpsychopathic individuals tend to utilize individuals with scores greater than 28 or 29 on the PCL-R (see as examples Hare & Forth, 1985; Newman & Schmitt, 1998; Newman, Schmitt, & Voss, 1997; Newman,

Wallace, Schmitt, & Arnett, 1997)[2] and compare them with those "low" on psychopathic traits while omitting the middle scoring group. Any differences are attributable to the extreme groups and not to the many individuals with moderate scores. There is a burden then on the clinician to ensure that these laboratory-based findings associated with "psychopathic" characteristics not be imputed to an individual for whom these differences have not been found.

Others have expressed concerns regarding the diagnosis of psychopathy and its implications and applications within the courts both in Canada (Zinger & Forth, 1998) and in the United States (Edens, 2001, 2006; Edens, Buffington-Vollum, Keilen, Roskamp, & Anthony, 2005). John Edens (2001) cites two inappropriate applications: one in which the PCL-R was entered as evidence for institutional violence, thus arguing for the death penalty; and the other using the absence of psychopathy (sociopathic tendencies) as evidence of innocence in a case of sexual abuse. Edens and colleagues (Edens, Colwell, Desforges, & Fernandez, 2005) found that among laypersons, introducing a diagnosis of psychopathy significantly increased the likelihood of support for the death penalty. Their findings were sufficiently stark that they recommended not introducing psychopathy into capital murder trials because of the potential for prejudicial treatment of the accused.

The critical issue in the use of psychopathy within forensic samples is to determine where the fulcrum lies that balances the utility of psychopathic traits against the possible misuses of the construct of psychopathy. Taken together, it is our opinion that the utility of the construct of psychopathy within forensic populations is limited. It is likely best used to explain the behavior of a small number of high-risk offenders, recalcitrant in their antisocial behavior and unresponsive to intervention. Psychopathy offers a potential biological perspective that when coupled with social-cognitive theory provides a reasonable explanation of the individual's behavior.

The use of psychopathic traits in risk assessment is ultimately up to the individual clinician's discretion. In our opinion, empirical advances during the past decade would serve to dampen exuberant statements that have been made regarding the centrality of the construct of psychopathy to the assessment of violence (Hart, 1998b; Salekin et al., 1996). We are of the opinion that it is not necessary to measure the construct of psychopathy to conduct a comprehensive assessment of violence risk. If as a clinician you choose to speak to the issue of psychopathic traits within the assessment of risk, then at the present time both research and practice would

---

[2]We recognize that not all neurophysiological studies use a cutoff score of 30 (see Intrator et al., 1997, who used a cutoff score of 25); however, this only serves to complicate the ability to infer underlying neurological performance with psychopathy.

indicate that you would use one of the PCL instruments. In our opinion, it is not acceptable to utilize a diagnosis of antisocial personality disorder as a proxy for a diagnosis of psychopathy as the literature indicates that there will be an overclassification and the two constructs are not the same (Hare, Hart, & Harpur, 1991; Hart & Hare, 1989). Nor is it acceptable to utilize a self-report instrument (e.g., MMPI, PAI, or a psychopathy-specific self-report instrument) as a proxy to inform on the diagnosis of psychopathy (Hare, 1985). The use of these instruments may inform the clinician on the pattern of antisocial behavior which is useful in violence risk assessment. Further, the use of one of the PCL instruments should only be undertaken after formal training or initially practiced while under the supervision and training of someone qualified to score the instrument. You will need more knowledge and training than is provided in the manual (Hare, 2003) to ethically administer and be adequately prepared to score and defend the use of psychopathy under cross-examination.

CONCLUSION

This review of risk factors indicates that individuals who develop an antisocial or criminal behavior pattern are more prone to perpetrate violence regardless of whether that risk for violence is general or specific (sexual or spousal) or if they have associated mental health issues. The general proclivity for antisocial behavior appears to support the manifestation of interpersonally intrusive and violent behavior. This may in fact explain what has been a long-standing relationship between psychopathy and violence. The risk for specific violence such as sexual or spousal violence is further elevated with risk factors specific to these types of violence. With this review complete, the next chapter considers the various types of risk appraisal instruments that have been more broadly validated through publication in peer-reviewed journals.

CHAPTER 3

■   ■   ■

RISK APPRAISAL INSTRUMENTS

After our explanation of the advancement of risk assessment (Chapter 1) and a review of the most significant risk factors for violence (Chapter 2), we now move into a review of a number of the more prominent risk appraisal instruments for violence assessment. These include examples of actuarial instruments that contain primarily static risk factors, structured professional judgment (SPJ) instruments, and dynamic–actuarial instruments. Each of these instruments has been shown to predict specific and often multiple types of violence. We have classified the instruments into those that predict nonsexual violence, those that were developed to predict general recidivism but have also been shown to predict violence, those that predict sexual violence, and those that predict spousal violence. We provide a general review of each instrument and provide as much detail as possible as to the items and scoring, though we are limited on some instruments due to copyright issues. Then we provide a summary of the validity findings within varying studies and samples. This information will be valuable when it comes time to choose the most appropriate instrument for your clientele, as well as when you prepare for testimony in legal proceedings. In addition, we comment on the literature that could speak to the *Daubert* guidelines for admissibility in court. Two points need to be stressed. First, recall that the *Daubert* guidelines are just that, guidelines, and they are not applied in all jurisdictions. Second, remember that it is up to the presiding judge, not the clinician or researcher, to determine if the guidelines are met. Our review, however, will help if you have to testify on these guidelines.

The instruments chosen for review in this chapter do not represent all valid violence risk appraisal instruments. In recent years there has been a proliferation of these types of instruments. Our general criteria for inclusion were that the instrument had to predict violence and had to have a track record within the peer-reviewed literature. Noninclusion of an instrument is not a reflection of our confidence in it. We have also included brief reviews of some instruments we think hold promise over time.

As we consider a number of risk assessment instruments, it is important to note that research articles are not free of bias. We don't suggest that data have been fudged or researchers have done anything unethical. Yet what we know from bias research tells us that, at times, an author is heavily vested with years (if not an entire career) in an instrument, and thus has defenses raised for mediocre or poor outcomes. Similarly, researchers like to compare the relative predictive accuracy of different instruments and report the various AUCs or r's. In most instances statistical comparisons of the relative accuracy of the instruments are not made, and the reader is left with the impression that one instrument may be more accurate than another. For example, an AUC for one instrument may be reported as .68 and for another .72, leaving the impression that the latter instrument is "more accurate." In fact, for the average research sample there is no meaningful difference between the two statistics. Variations of this nature are to be expected and depend on a wide variety of influences such as the specific sample composition, the type of outcome considered, and the length of follow-up time, to mention only a few.

When considering the predictive validity of a risk appraisal instrument the key issue is the *preponderance of evidence*: overall, what does the research indicate? Reviewing the literature as a whole and assessing trends is typical for most consumers of research. Meta-analyses (combining the outcomes from many different research reports) have become one method for researchers to *research the research*. Meta-analyses permit researchers to convert outcomes from many different studies into the same metric and average the effect size. With increasingly more outcome studies becoming available, meta-analyses have been more frequently reported in the literature. It is important to note that an individual study will not make or break an instrument; rather, it is the preponderance of evidence that really matters.

The methodology of a research effort is very important to the outcome and predictive accuracy of risk assessment instruments. For example, most follow-up studies contain individuals with varying lengths of follow-up time in the community (from several months to several years). This is done to retain as may individuals as possible within the study sample. However, some researchers have found that the predictive accuracy of instruments improves when a constant follow-up period is employed (Harris et al., 2003; Langton et al., 2007). A similar improvement was shown when only assessment protocols with no missing risk factors are included in the analysis (Harris et al., 2003). Additionally, formal training and experience in the administration of risk assessment instruments have been shown to improve the relationship between an actuarial instrument such as the LSI-R and the outcome of recidivism (Flores, Lowenkamp, Holsinger, & Latessa, 2006).

Outcomes of research with assessment instruments typically include recidivism or no recidivism. It is important to note that what these instruments are predicting is the relationship of the instrument with *known* or *detected* recidivism. There are offenders who reoffend but whose offenses are not detected. These occurrences serve to reduce the rates of recidivism reported as well as to render the instrument potentially less accurate. This means that while we measure outcome as dichotomous (reoffended vs. did not reoffend) actual outcome is trichotomous and includes those who did reoffend but were not detected. Leistico et al. (2008) argue convincingly that as follow-up time lengthens more offenders move from the reoffended but undetected group to the detected group and that this is what accounts for the difference in predictive effect size between shorter follow-up periods, and longer follow-up periods with the latter having greater effect sizes.

As you will see in the following pages, much research completed on risk assessment instruments is retrospective, because of the time lag between administering an instrument and waiting a matter of years for follow-up data on recidivism. Retrospective methods have appeal because instruments can be coded from file and the outcome is already known. However, retrospective studies are not the "gold standard" though they do help to provide evidence for the validity of the instruments.

This chapter focuses on clinician-rated instruments. We do note that self-report measures can play an important role in the assessment enterprise. Contrary to conventional thinking that offender self-report cannot be trusted, there is ample evidence to the contrary (Kroner & Loza, 2001; Mills, Kroner, & Hemmati, 2004; Mills, Loza, & Kroner, 2003). Of particular note is a meta-analysis conducted by Glenn Walters (2006) wherein he compares the effect size (correlations) between five commonly used clinician-rated risk appraisal instruments with self-report instruments in the prediction of criminal justice outcomes (i.e., recidivism, disciplinary infractions, violence). Clinician-rated instruments were superior to self-report until a secondary analysis that compared these two procedures on content-relevant self-report measures—that is, those self-report instruments developed specifically for the criminal offender and antisocial client with item content that contains criminal offending and antisocial features. At this point clinician-rated assessments were not superior but equal to self-report assessments. Further analysis showed that each method added to the other in the prediction of the outcome, leading to the conclusion that self-report assessments do have information to add to the risk assessment enterprise. Our own research indicates that self-report is effective in predicting outcome (Mills et al., 2004; Mills, Loza, & Kroner, 2003); however, we recognize that in most jurisdictions and circumstances self-report will at best only be an adjunct in the prediction of violence. Decision-making bodies rely on the professional's opinion based upon the professional's assessment using risk appraisal instruments that are clinician-rated. It has been our experience that self-report measures are typically a unidirectional contributor to the assessment process: they can buttress a negative (high-risk) assessment but rarely support a positive (low-risk) assessment because of the assumption of a response bias (socially desirable responding).

Multicollinearity of Risk Factors

One phenomena that is consistent in the risk assessment enterprise is the multicollinearity of risk factors. Simply put, individual risk factors tend to correlate with other risk factors. Individuals who score high on one set of risk factors tend to score high on other sets of risk factors. Those with a history of criminal behavior often have a history of substance abuse and a history of criminal associations. Each of these three areas contains risk factors, but in large samples they also tend to have moderate-to-strong intercorrelations. This means that risk factors tend to add only incrementally to each other in the overall prediction of violence. Because it is unwieldy to include all possible risk factors in any risk assessment, as there are literally dozens of factors that are related to criminal and violent behavior, assessments therefore tend to choose either rationally or empirically from among groups of variables when establishing a risk assessment instrument (Hilton et al., 2004; Quinsey et al., 2006; Webster, Eaves, Douglas, & Wintrup. 1995). This inevitably means that some risk factors that have been shown to be related to violence are not included in risk assessment schemes, and while there is much similarity among the risk assessment instruments, there are also differences.

One unique empirical example of multicollinearity was a study that took all of the items from four prominent risk assessment instruments, 101 in total, and placed them in an empty coffee can (Kroner et al., 2005). Thirteen items were selected randomly without replacement and added to the variable of prior incarcerations (a criminal history variable common to most assessment instruments). Four randomly derived "instruments" were created and compared with the original four assessment instruments in terms of their predictive validity. No differences were found. A factor analysis of the same four original risk assessment instruments was conducted on 1,614 cases. Four factor-derived scales were identified, after which it was determined that these factor-derived scales were also no better at predicting recidivism than the randomly derived instruments. This finding is not surprising because of the presence of multicollinearity between risk assessment factors. Once enough variables (in this case 14) that are related to recidivism have been sampled, the association with recidivism is robust. As noted above, the method of item selection explains in part why there are differences in absolute accuracy of instruments. Multicollinearity explains why, despite the differences, in practice instruments do not consistently differ in a statistically meaningful way from each other in predictive accuracy. This may also lead clinicians who employ clinical over-rides to inflate an individual's risk to reoffend. That is to say that the factors included in the instrument are likely correlated with the other factors the clinician is using to adjust (increase) risk estimates—said another way, the predictive information in the additional risk factors may have already been accounted for by those risk factors already considered.

INSTRUMENTS SPECIFICALLY DEVELOPED TO PREDICT NONSEXUAL VIOLENCE

Violence Risk Appraisal Guide

The Violence Risk Appraisal Guide (VRAG; Harris et al., 1993; Quinsey et al., 1998, 2006) was developed retrospectively on a sample of forensic psychiatric inpatients and individuals referred for competency assessment. The selection of items was a purely statistical exercise with serious violence as the outcome of interest. The 12 items of the VRAG (see Table 3.1) were selected according to the ability of each item to discriminate between violent recidivists and nonrecidivists. A stepwise discriminant function analysis was used to determine which items had the strongest predictive power. Each item was then given a weighting of +1 or −1 for every plus or minus 5% differ-ence from the mean recidivism rate (base rate) of 31%. This is a weighted system and resulted in the total score of the VRAG ranging from −26 to

TABLE 3.1. Items of the Violence Risk Appraisal Guide

- Lived with both parents to the age of 16
- Elementary school maladjustment
- History of alcohol problems
- Marital status
- Criminal history score for nonviolent offenses
- Failure on conditional release
- Age at index offense
- Victim injury
- Female victim
- DSM diagnosis of any personality disorder
- DSM diagnosis of schizophrenia
- PCL-R or CATS

38, with higher scores reflecting a greater likelihood of violent reoffending. Research that has compared a variety of weighting methods showed no improvement in predictive accuracy of a risk assessment instrument with weighted systems (Grann & Langstrom, 2007).

Interrater correlations for the VRAG items are above .80 and kappas are above .70 (Rice, Harris, & Cormier, 1992; Rice, Harris, & Quinsey, 1990). Kroner and Mills (2001) found intraclass correlation to equal .95. Rice and Harris (1997) reported interrater reliability of the VRAG to be .90. Three items (separation from parents before age 16, elementary school adjustment, and Psychopathy Checklist—Revised [PCL-R; Hare, 1991, 2003]) refer to development issues; five items are based on current and past offenses (age at index offense, victim injury, alcohol abuse, gender of victim, history of nonviolent offenses); the other four items are diagnosis of personality disorder, diagnosis of schizophrenia, marital status, and failure on prior conditional release. More recently the Childhood and Adolescent Taxon Scale (CATS; Quinsey, Harris, et al., 2006) can be substituted for the PCL-R, which significantly reduces the time necessary to score the instrument.

Studies of the predictive accuracy of the VRAG have shown the instrument to predict violent recidivism among both psychiatric and nonpsychiatric samples (see Table 3.2 for a list of relevant outcome studies). Psychiatric patients followed for periods of 2 and 10 years were assessed using the VRAG, which produced accuracy estimates in the moderate-to-high range (AUCs of .68 and .77) (Grann, Belfrage, & Tengstrom, 2000; Rice & Harris, 1995). Loza and Dhaliwal (1997) studied the VRAG with correctional offenders and found that it was able to distinguish between violent and nonviolent offenders. The VRAG has also been shown to be a strong predictor of future violence among released psychiatric patients with a diagnosis of mental retardation (Quinsey, Book, & Skilling, 2004). In this study the VRAG was scored using the CATS instead of the PCL-R. The accuracy of the VRAG in predicting violence in the original sample as represented by AUC was .76. Recall that the AUC is a statistic of receiver operating characteristic analysis and it represents the likelihood that a randomly chosen recidivist would have a higher score than a randomly chosen nonrecidivist. In this instance the AUC of .76 means that a randomly chosen recidivist would have a higher score than a nonrecidivist 76% of the time. AUCs that exceed .70 are considered large effect sizes. Similarly, the VRAG predicted general (AUC = .67) and violent (AUC = .60) recidivism in a sample of violent offenders with an average of a 2-year follow-up period (Kroner & Mills, 2001).

The VRAG was examined among civilly committed psychiatric patients by Harris, Rice, and Camilleri (2004) using item approximations based on the MacArthur Violence Risk Assessment Study (Monahan et al., 2001).

TABLE 3.2. Outcomes for Studies Using the VRAG

Study	Sample description				Criterion and follow-up	Outcome
	Participants	Sex	Jurisdiction	Race		
Harris, Rice, & Quinsey (1993)	Forensic inpatients	Male	Canada	Mixed	Retrospective, 82 months	Criminal charges for violence AUC = .76
Rice & Harris (1995)	Sex offenders	Male	Canada	Not reported	Retrospective, 10 years	Violent recidivism AUC = .77
Grann, Belfrage, & Tengstrom (2000)[a]	Forensic psychiatric	Male	Sweden	Not reported	Retrospective, 2 years	Violent reconviction AUC = .68
Kroner & Mills (2001)	Correctional	Male	Canada	Predominantly white	Predictive, 2 years	Convictions for violence AUC = .60
Barbaree, Seto, Langton, & Peacock (2001)	Correctional sex offenders	Male	Canada	Mixed	Retrospective, 4.5 years	Violent offenses AUC = .69; sexual offenses AUC = .61
Harris, Rice, & Cormier (2002)	Forensic inpatients	Male	Canada	Mixed	Predictive, 5 years	Criminal charges for violence AUC = .80
Harris et al. (2003)	1. Forensic inpatients 2. Correctional psychiatric 3. Correctional psychiatric	Male Male Male	Canada Canada Canada	Mixed Mixed Mixed	Predictive, 3 years Predictive, 3 years Predictive, 3 years	Violent offenses AUC = .77 Violent offenses AUC = .70 Violent offenses AUC = .70
Harris, Rice, & Camilleri (2004)[b]	Hospital inpatients	Mixed	United States	Mixed	Predictive, 20 weeks	Self-reported violence AUC = .72; men AUC = .71; women AUC = .73
Quinsey, Book, & Skilling (2004)	Mentally retarded psychiatric patients	Male	Canada	Mixed	Predictive, 15 months	Any violent incident r = .32, AUC = .69

(continued)

TABLE 3.2. (*continued*)

| Study | Sample description | | | Criterion and follow-up | Outcome |
	Participants	Sex	Jurisdiction	Race		
Mills, Jones, & Kroner (2005)	Correctional	Male	Canada	Predominantly white	Predictive, 3 years	Convictions for violence $r = .26$
Douglas, Yeomans, & Boer (2005)	Correctional	Male	Canada	Predominantly white	Retrospective, 7.7 years	Violent reoffending AUC = .79
Langton et al. (2007)	Sexual offenders	Male	Canada	Not reported	Retrospective, 3 years	Violent reoffending AUC = .73
Gray, Fitzgerald, Taylor, MacCulloch, & Snowden (2007)	Offenders with serious mental illness	Mixed	United Kingdom	Not reported	File review-based prospective	Offenders with intellectual disabilities: general reconviction AUC = .74, violent reconviction AUC = .73. Offenders with serious mental illness: general reconviction AUC = .73, violent reconviction AUC = .74

[a]Two items of the VRAG (items 7 and 11) could not be scored.

[b]Ten-item VRAG adapted from MacArthur Study data (see Monahan et al., 2001).

This modified VRAG produced AUCs of .72 and .70 for violence within 20-weeks and 50-weeks, respectively. In a subsequent analysis of the same data with a similar but not exact item approximation, Edens, Skeem, and Douglas (2006) analyzed the incremental validity of these instruments and found that the predictive accuracy of the VRAG without the PCL: SV was degraded. This was not inconsistent with the original findings of Monahan et al. (2001), who concluded that the PCL: SV was the strongest of over 100 potential risk factors.

A study by Wagdy Loza and colleagues (Loza, Villeneuve, & Loza-Fanous, 2002) within a sample of correctional offenders found the VRAG to be predictive of reoffense and any failure on release, though not so for violence in particular. It should be recognized that the base rate for violence in the study was only 12.9%, which is fairly low and may explain the lack of predictive efficacy. More important, however, was the finding that when the scores were categorized into low, moderate, and high groupings there was little differentiation between the high and moderate groups. In a similar study of the VRAG with a correctional offender sample Mills, Jones, and Kroner (2005) found that the recidivism rates within the nine risk bins of the VRAG were not consistent with those rates found in the original sample of scale development. In fact, there were two instances in which a bin of higher expected recidivism actually had a lower rate of recidivism than the bin that preceded it. This finding sparked further investigation into the relationship of the VRAG items with the outcome of violent recidivism within a correctional sample (Mills et al., 2007). The results showed that only 5 of the 12 VRAG items distinguished between violent recidivists and the remaining participants. The correlation therefore within this sample was being driven by the items that were related to violence while the other variables did not contribute to the relationship. However, those items not related to violence could contribute to overall score fluctuation between the predictive bins.

Harris et al. (2002) found that the VRAG did not distinguish between recidivists and nonrecidivists in a subsample of female forensic patients. Cross-validation studies on international samples showed moderate-to-high predictive accuracy rates. In a Swedish sample of mentally disordered offenders, the AUC of the VRAG was lower in absolute terms (AUC = .68; Grann et al., 2000); however, in a study conducted in the United Kingdom, Gray, Fitzgerald, Taylor, MacCulloch, and Snowden (2007) found high predictive accuracy for violence (AUC from .73 to .74).

HCR-20

The HCR-20, originally developed by Webster et al. (1995), derives its name from the type and number of items that the instrument contains: 10 historical items, 5 clinical items, and 5 risk management items (see Table

3.3). Very soon afterward a revision was published that served to clarify the administration and coding procedures based upon feedback from the initial release (Webster et al., 1997). The HCR-20 falls into the category of an SPJ assessment instrument.

The 20 items of the HCR-20 are scored 0, 1, or 2. A score of zero means the available information contraindicates the presence of the item, a score of 1 means the available information suggests the possible presence of the item, and a score of 2 means the available information indicates the presence of the item.

The HCR-20's concurrent validity and interrater agreement has been demonstrated among offenders (intraclass correlation [ICC] = .82; Douglas & Webster, 1999) and civilly committed patients (ICC = .80; Douglas, Ogloff, Nicholls, & Grant, 1999). Elsewhere ICCs from .80 to .88 among offenders with serious mental illness have been found (Gray et al., 2007). Kroner and Mills (2001) reported an ICC of .85 in a sample of correctional offenders.

Douglas and Ogloff (2003) compared the accuracy of violence risk estimates using HCR-20 scores and the subsequent descriptive categories of low, moderate, and high risk between those cases in which raters had high confidence and those cases in which the raters had low confidence in the "certainty or reliance or trust about the correctness of the rating." Those ratings with comparatively high confidence were in fact more accurate than those ratings that had low confidence.

TABLE 3.3. Items of the HCR-20

Historical	Clinical	Risk management
H1 Previous violence	C1 Lack of insight	R1 Plans lack feasibility
H2 Young age at first violent incident	C2 Negative attitudes	R2 Exposure to destabilizers
H3 Relationship instability	C3 Active symptoms of major mental illness	R3 Lack of personal support
H4 Employment problems	C4 Impulsivity	R4 Noncompliance with remediation attempts
H5 Substance use problems	C5 Unresponsive to treatment	R5 Stress
H6 Major mental illness		
H7 Psychopathy		
H8 Early maladjustment		
H9 Personality disorder		
H10 Prior supervision failure		

A retrospective study with civilly committed psychiatric inpatients in Canada demonstrated good predictive qualities of the HCR-20 and its subscales in predicting criminal violence: HCR-20 total AUC = .80, H10 subscale AUC = .78, C5 subscale AUC = .63, and R5 subscale AUC = .74. Predictive validity of the HCR-20 within an offender sample has also been demonstrated (Douglas, Yeomans, & Boer, 2005; Kroner & Mills, 2001). The HCR-20 has also been shown to differentiate between offenders who were violent in prison and those who were not violent (Belfrage, Fransson, & Strand, 2000). Other research with offenders has shown the HCR-20 to have a moderate effect size when predicting minor institutional misconduct (AUC = .68) and a small effect size when predicting major misconduct (AUC = .57). The historical portion has been shown to be predictive of future violence in mentally disordered offenders (Grann et al., 2000). A retrospective study in the United Kingdom that followed up released secure facility psychiatric patients found the HCR-20 to be predictive of readmission, self-report/collateral reports of violence, and general reoffending (Dolan & Khawaja, 2004), despite the fact that the PCL-R was omitted from the instrument. Table 3.4 lists a number of relevant studies examining the HCR-20.

Male and female psychiatric patients were compared on their HCR-20 scores, and no significant differences were found between their overall and subscale scores (de Vogel & de Ruiter, 2005). The same study examined the predictive accuracy of the HCR-20 with subsequent violence. Among male patients the HCR-20 was accurate (AUC = .88), whereas for female patients the accuracy was not significantly different from chance (AUC = .59). Overall risk judgments of low, moderate, and high were, however, more encouragingly accurate (males, AUC = .91 and females, AUC = .86). In another retrospective study (Nicholls, Ogloff, & Douglas, 2004) the HCR-20 demonstrated similar accuracy with both male and female psychiatric patients when predicting any violence (male, AUC = .72; female, AUC = .77) and when predicting violent crime (male, AUC = .75; female, AUC = .80). Gender differences were evident in the strength of the relationship between the HC-15[1] and inpatient violence as well as the mean score of the HCR-20. Moderate relationships were found between the HC-15 scores and both physical inpatient violence and any inpatient violence for women (r = .18 and .32, respectively), whereas there were no significant relationships between inpatient violence and the HC-15 for men. Contrary to the de Vogel and de Ruiter (2005) study, significant differences were found between male inpatient (M = 20.4) and female inpatient (M = 16.8) HCR-20 scores.

Within a female correctional sample HCR-20 scores showed excellent interrater agreement (ICC = .94) and were more strongly correlated to Fac-

---

[1]Only the historical and clinical items were used for the prediction of inpatient violence.

TABLE 3.4. Outcomes for Studies Using the HCR-20

Study	Sample description				Criterion and follow-up	Outcome
	Participants	Sex	Jurisdiction	Race		
Douglas, Ogloff, Nicholls, & Grant (1999)	Civilly committed psychiatric inpatients	Mixed	Canada	Predominantly white	Retrospective, 21 months	Criminal violence HCR-20; total AUC = .80
Kroner & Mills (2001)	Correctional	Male	Canada	Predominantly white	Predictive, 2 years	Convictions for violence AUC = .62; any reoffense AUC = .65
Gray et al. (2003)	Psychiatric inpatients	Mixed	United Kingdom	Predominantly white	Predictive, 3 months	Inpatient physical aggression AUC = .81
Gray et al. (2004)	Secure psychiatric	Mixed	United Kingdom	Predominantly white	Retrospective, 6 years	Any criminal offense AUC = .61; serious criminal offense (violence) AUC = .56.
Dolan & Khawaja (2004)	Secure psychiatric	Male	United Kingdom	Predominantly white	Retrospective, 5 years	Readmission AUC = .85; self/collateral reports of violence AUC = .76; reoffending AUC = .76
Nicholls, Ogloff, & Douglas (2004)	Involuntary hospitalized psychiatric patients	Male	Canada	Predominantly white	Retrospective, 2 years	Inpatient physical violence (HC-15) AUC = .56; community violence AUC = .73; violent crime AUC = .75
Nicholls, Ogloff, & Douglas (2004)	Involuntary hospitalized psychiatric patients	Female	Canada	Predominantly white	Retrospective, 2 years	Inpatient physical violence (HC-15) AUC = .62; Community violence AUC = .66; violent crime AUC = .80
de Vogel & de Ruiter (2005)	Forensic psychiatric hospital	Mixed	Netherlands	Predominantly white	Retrospective, 6.7 years	Combined inpatient and community violence: male AUC = .88; female AUC = .59

Study	Sample	Gender	Country	Ethnicity	Design	Results
Douglas, Yeomans, & Boer (2005)	Correctional	Male	Canada	Predominantly white	Retrospective, 7.7 years	Violent reoffending AUC = .82
Stadtland et al. (2005)	Correctional sex offenders	Male	Germany	Not reported	Retrospective, 9 years	Violent offenses AUC = .65
Dahle (2006)	Correctional	Male	Germany	Not reported	Retrospective, Greater than 10 years	Reimprisonment r = .31; violent crime r = .31
Gray, Fitzgerald, Taylor, MacCulloch, & Snowden (2007)	Offenders with serious mental illness	Mixed	United Kingdom	Not reported	File review-based prospective	Offenders with intellectual disabilities: general reconviction AUC = .81; violent reconviction AUC = .79. Offenders with serious mental illness: general reconviction AUC = .68, violent reconviction AUC = .68

tor 2 (antisocial lifestyle) than to Factor 1 (personality characteristics) of the PCL-R (Warren et al., 2005). Cautious use of the HCR-20 with women is recommended (Nicholls et al., 2004).

Sex Offender Risk Appraisal Guide

The Sex Offender Risk Appraisal Guide (SORAG; Quinsey et al., 2006) was developed to predict violent re-offending (both nonsexual and sexual violence) among sex offenders. In that sense it differs from other instruments developed for use among sex offenders, which focus on the prediction of sexual violence exclusively. This is why the SORAG, an instrument for use with sex offenders, is contained in this section—its primary objective was the prediction of any violence among sex offenders. The SORAG is a 14-item instrument that overlaps considerably with the VRAG (see Table 3.5 for a list of the items). Notable differences are the inclusion of items such as convictions for previous sexual offenses, a history of sex offenses against male children or adults, and phallometrically determined sexual deviance. The instrument has been shown to demonstrate predictive validity when used with correctional sex offenders and sex offenders within forensic psychiatric settings. A list of relevant studies are contained in Table 3.6. Instructions on scoring and the interpretive predictive categories are reported in Quinsey, et al. (2006).

TABLE 3.5. Items of the SORAG

- Lived with both biological parents to the age of 16
- Elementary school maladjustment
- History of alcohol problems
- Marital status
- Criminal history of nonviolent offenses
- Criminal history of violent offenses
- Convictions for previous sexual offenses
- History of sex offenses against girls under 14 years
- Failure on prior conditional release
- Age at index (current) offense
- DSM diagnosis of personality disorder
- DSM diagnosis for schizophrenia
- Any deviant sexual preference on a phallometric test
- Psychopathy

TABLE 3.6. Outcomes for Studies Using the SORAG

Study	Sample description				Criterion and follow-up	Outcome
	Participants	Sex	Jurisdiction	Race		
Barbaree, Seto, Langton, & Peacock (2001)	Correctional sex offenders	Male	Canada	Mixed	Retrospective, 4.5 years	Violent offense AUC = .73; sexual offense AUC = .70
Bartosh, Garby, Lewis, & Gray (2003)	Correctional sex offenders	Male	United States	Mixed	Retrospective, 5 years	Sexual offense AUC = .58; violent offense AUC = .72; sexual/violent offense AUC = .64
Harris et al. (2003)	1. Forensic inpatients	Male	Canada	Mixed	Predictive, 3 years	Violent offenses AUC = .77; sexual offense AUC = .71
	2. Correctional psychiatric	Male	Canada	Mixed	Predictive, 3 years	Violent offenses AUC = .71; sexual offense AUC = .62
	3. Correctional psychiatric	Male	Canada	Mixed	Predictive, 3 years	Violent offenses AUC = .69; Sexual offense AUC = .59
Ducro & Pham (2006)	Hospitalized sex offenders	Male	Belgium	Not reported	Retrospective, 4.2 years	Sexual offence AUC = .64; nonsexual violence AUC = .72.
Langton et al. (2007)	Sexual offenders	Male	Canada	Not reported	Retrospective, 3 years	Violent reoffending AUC = .74
Knight & Thornton (2007)	Correctional sex offenders	Male	United States	Predominantly white	Retrospective, fixed 3, 10, and 15 years	Sexual reoffending 3-year AUC = .67; 10-year AUC = .67
Kingston, Yates, Firestone, Babchishin, & Bradford (2008)	1. Sex offenders 2. Psychiatric hospital outpatients	Male	Canada	Not reported	Retrospective, 11.4 years	Sexual offense AUC = .77 Violent and sexual offense AUC = .76

Violence Risk Scale

The Violence Risk Scale (VRS; Wong & Gordon, 2006) was developed specifically to measure change in risk associated with a change resulting from treatment. This instrument does not have a strong track record in the peer-reviewed literature but has excellent potential and falls within the category of a truly dynamic–actuarial instrument. The authors of the VRS report that their theoretical orientation in the development of the instrument was based on the psychology of criminal conduct (Andrews & Bonta, 2003), the principles of effective correctional treatment (Andrews & Bonta, 2003), and the Transtheoretical Model of Change (Prochaska & DiClemente, 1984). Given the focus on measuring change, dynamic items on the VRS outnumber the static items 20 to 6.

The six static variables of the VRS include current age, age of first violent conviction, number of juvenile convictions, violence throughout the lifespan, prior release failures/escapes, and stability of family upbringing. The 20 dynamic variables include violent lifestyle, criminal personality, criminal attitude, work ethic, criminal peers, interpersonal aggression, emotional regulation/control, violence during institutionalization, weapon use, insight into violence, mental illness, substance abuse, stability of relationships, community support, released to high-risk situations, violence cycle, impulsivity, cognitive distortion, compliance with supervision, and the security level of releasing institution. All variables on the VRS are rated on a 4-point Likert scale (0, 1, 2, or 3), with the higher numbers representing a greater presence of the construct being measured. Risk reduction is also predicated on a progression through the stages of change with the exception that a change in a variable for a client moving from precontemplation to contemplation would not be considered a change in risk.

Interrater reliabilities of the VRS were approximated using intraclass correlation coefficients (r = .92 and .97) and Pearson correlations (r = .87) and found to be quite acceptable. Cronback alpha coefficients, a measure of scale internal consistency, were found to be acceptable: VRS total = .93, dynamic items = .94, and static items = .69. Intercorrelations of the VRS with other risk-related instruments are considered moderate to strong: VRS Static with PCL-R r = .61, GSIR r = .71, LSI-R r = .64; VRS Dynamic with PCL-R r = .83, GSIR r = .55, LSI-R r = .88. The predictive accuracy of the VRS for all 918 participants over an average follow-up period of 4.4 years was good (AUC = .75) and consistent with the performance of other similar instruments. Another published study used the VRS within a sample of secure psychiatric inpatients scoring it retrospectively and examined the outcome of institutional violence (Dolan & Fullam, 2007). The VRS was found to be very strongly correlated (r = .92) with the HCR-20 and had the same level of predictive accuracy (VRS: AUC = .713; HCR-20: AUC = .715).

INSTRUMENTS DEVELOPED TO PREDICT GENERAL REOFFENDING THAT ALSO PREDICT NONSEXUAL VIOLENCE

Level of Service Inventory—Revised

The Level of Service Inventory—Revised (LSI-R; Andrews & Bonta, 1995) is a 54-item instrument that assesses 10 areas (see Table 3.7) relevant to criminal history and criminogenic need (those areas of personal/social function that can change and are related to criminal recidivism). The instrument contains items that are both historical/static as well as items that are dynamic in nature as they have the potential to change over the course of months and years (Mills, Kroner, & Hemmati, 2003). The instrument was developed to assess the risk for supervision failure among offenders serving sentences of less than 2 years in the province of Ontario. The LSI-R was primarily developed with general recidivism as an outcome. However, research has shown that the scores are significantly related to outcome, with an accuracy similar to instruments developed for the exclusive assessment of violence. Violent prisoners score higher on the LSI-R than nonviolent prisoners (Hollin & Palmer, 2003; Loza & Simourd, 1994), which speaks to the level of risk as well as the need for greater intervention to manage that risk (greater criminogenic needs).

The LSI-R was developed from a social learning perspective; thus, the instrument measures areas of personal history and interaction with others. Validity studies with samples similar to the initial validation sample show

TABLE 3.7. Areas Assessed by the LSI-R Using Static and Potentially Dynamic Items

Area Assessed	Static	Potentially Dynamic
1. Criminal history	√	
2. Education/employment	√	√
3. Financial		√
4. Family/marital	√	√
5. Accommodation		√
6. Leisure/recreation		√
7. Companions		√
8. Alcohol/drugs	√	√
9. Emotional/personal	√	√
10. Attitude/orientation		√

that higher LSI-R scores have been associated with parole failure and a return to custody (Bonta & Motiuk, 1990; Motiuk, Bonta, & Andrews, 1986), as well as with institutional misconduct (Bonta, 1989; Bonta & Motiuk, 1987). Other studies employing the LSI-R have shown similar evidence of predictive validity. Loza and Simourd (1994) reported on the validity of the LSI-R with Canadian offenders sentenced to 2 or more years in prison and found that the LSI-R total and its component subscales were related to psychopathic traits and actuarial risk. Simourd and Malcolm (1998) found the LSI-R to evidence concurrent validity and internal consistency within a sample of incarcerated sex offenders. Table 3.8 provides a list of relevant outcome studies.

Dahle (2006) reported good interrater agreement on retrospectively coded files in a sample of German offenders (ICC = .91). Correlations with reoffense (r = .29) and violent crime (r = .23) over a 10-year follow-up period were consistent with other correlates of recidivism such as the HCR-20 and PCL-R.

The LSI-R and a variant of the LSI-R have also been shown to be predictive among native and young offender samples, respectively (Bonta, LaPrairie, & Wallace-Capretta, 1997; Jung & Rawana, 1999). For example, among the aboriginal offenders (North American Native) the risk factors of alcohol/drugs, attitude, criminal history, financial, peers, and employment were all associated with recidivism. Traditional risk factors that were not related to recidivism for aboriginal offenders included family/marital problems, emotional, mental ability, and academic/vocational problems. However, the overall score of the risk/needs instrument was related to recidivism. In general, then, most traditional risk factors are associated with recidivism and have the benefit of identifying points for intervention.

Fass, Heilbrun, Dematteo, and Fretz (2008) examined the relative accuracy of the LSI-R between ethnic groups. There were some differences noted in the overall level of accuracy in predicting rearrest. AUC for Caucasian offenders was .55, for African American offenders was .61, and for Hispanic offenders was .54. This is somewhat unexpected in that the LSI-R was developed on a predominantly white Canadian sample. There was a base rate of 21% over the 12-month follow-up period. The relatively low base rate is likely due to the brief follow-up period. The results of this study with respect to informing on ethnic differences should be cautiously considered given that the LSI-R's accuracy was lower than most other cross-validation studies and its accuracy for the Caucasian sample was lower than another ethnic group. Another study reported that the internal consistency estimates and intercorrelations among the subscales of the LSI-R were quite variable for both African American and Hispanic offenders (Schlager & Simourd, 2007). In addition, the LSI-R scores were correlated with rearrest and reconviction for African Americans and Hispanics, but only reconviction among

TABLE 3.8. Outcomes for Studies Using the LSI-R

Study	Sample description				Criterion and follow-up	Outcome
	Participants	Sex	Jurisdiction	Race		
Lowenkamp, Holsinger, & Latessa (2001)	Correctional	Male and female	United States	Near equal mix of white and African American	Predictive, 1.6 years	Reincarceration: males $r = .22$, females $r = .37$
Kroner & Mills (2001)	Correctional	Male	Canada	Predominantly white	Predictive, 2 years	Convictions for violence AUC = .66; Any reoffense AUC = .69
Girard & Wormith (2004)	Correctional	Male	Canada	Predominantly white	Predictive, 2½ years	General reoffense AUC = .73; Violent reoffense AUC = .68
Simourd (2004)	Correctional	Male	Canada	Predominantly white	Predictive, 15 months	Rearrest $r = .44$, reincarceration $r = .50$
Mills, Jones, & Kroner (2005)	Correctional	Male	Canada	Predominantly white	Predictive, 3 years	Convictions for any reoffense $r = .39$
Dahle (2006)	Correctional	Male	Germany	Not reported	Retrospective, > 10 years	Reimprisonment $r = .29$, violent crime $r = .23$
Hollin & Palmer (2006)	Correctional	Male	England	Not reported	Predictive, 13 months	Reconviction $r = .25$
Palmer & Hollin (2007)	Correctional	Female	England	Predominantly white	Predictive, 2.5 years	Reconviction $r = .53$
Schlager & Simourd (2007)	Community correctional	Male	United States	African American and Hispanic	Predictive, 2 years	African American: rearrest $r = $ ns, reconviction $r = .11$. Hispanic rearrest $r = $ ns, reconviction $r = $ ns

(continued)

83

TABLE 3.8. (*continued*)

Study	Sample description				Criterion and follow-up	Outcome
	Participants	Sex	Jurisdiction	Race		
Manchak, Skeem, & Douglas (2007)	Correctional	Male	United States	Predominantly white	Predictive, 1 year	Long-term offenders: general recidivism AUC = .73, violent recidivism AUC = .73. General offenders: general recidivism AUC = .66, violent recidivism AUC = .66
Fass, Heilbrun, Dematteo, & Fretz (2008)	Correctional	Male	United States	Mixed	Retrospective, 12 months	Caucasian AUC = .55, African American AUC = .61, Hispanic AUC = .54
Kelly & Welsh (2008)	Correctional-treated substance abusers	Male	United States	Not reported	Predictive, 15 months	Reincarceration (not reoffense) r = .25

African American offenders was significant over 2 years and the strength of that relationship was quite weak when compared with other studies. Other research has found that the LSI-R may both overclassify African Americans as high risk (identify as high risk but were successful) and underclassify Caucasians and Hispanics (identify as low risk those who failed) (Fass et al., 2008). These findings were considered preliminary but there was the suggestion that certain of the socioeconomic risk factors in the LSI-R may need to be reconsidered in light of possible racial differences. This may readily be dealt with by adjusting cutoff scores (renorming), or it may also require revisiting the measurement of those content areas.

One of the first studies to examine the LSI-R among female offenders was conducted by Christopher Lowenkamp and colleagues (Lowenkamp, Holsinger, & Latessa, 2001). They compared male and female offenders within the same study and examined the relationship of the LSI-R with the three different outcomes: successful program completion, absconding, and reincarceration. The strength of the relationship between the LSI-R and these outcome measures were quite similar for both men and women: successful program completion (males $r = .24$, females $r = .25$), absconding (males $r = .13$, females $r = .18$), and reincarceration (males $r = .22$, females $r = .37$). The rates of recidivism associated with varying ranges of scores were as follows: LSI-R scores 0–20 (males 29%, females 17%), LSI-R scores 21–30 (males 41%, females 31%), and LSI-R scores 31+ (males 58%, females 56%). The authors additionally sought to determine if a history of childhood abuse or race would add to the risk information in the LSI-R to predict the outcome of reincarceration. Neither variable added to the prediction of reincarceration in both the male and females samples.

An early self-report version of the original LSI was shown to correlate very well with three outcome measures among female offenders (Coulson, Ilacqua, Nutbrown, Giulekas, & Cudjoe, 1996). The point-biserial relationships were $r = .51$ for recidivism, $r = .53$ for parole failure, and $r = .45$ for halfway house failure. Similar results with a self-report LSI-R were found among female offenders who were serving longer sentences. Jean Folsom and Jill Atkinson (2007) found that after an average period of 6 years postrelease the LSI-R self-report was correlated significantly with outcome ($r = .30$). A study of female English prisoners found significant gender differences in the means of the various subscales of the LSI-R when compared with the male English counterparts (Palmer & Hollin, 2007). Specifically, men had more criminal history and greater leisure time deficits, whereas women had greater needs in the areas of family/marital, accommodation, drug/alcohol, emotional/personal, and antisocial companions.

The LSI-R contains items that are static and potentially dynamic (have the potential to change over time) (Mills, Kroner, & Hemmati, 2003). Some researchers suggest that for offenders serving long-term sentences it is appropriate to adjust some of the dynamic items to reflect their institutional functioning (Simourd, 2004). These adjusted scores have been shown to correlate with measures of recidivism over a 15-month follow-up period. One research effort on English prisoners compared LSI-R scores on entry to prison with LSI-R scores measured just prior to release (Hollin & Palmer, 2006; Hollin, Palmer, & Clark, 2003). In aggregate, the difference in the scores were statistically significant but small (LSI-R at intake = 21.98 and LSI-R at discharge = 21.25). The authors did not compare the two measures in predictive accuracy.

Statistical Information on Recidivism—Revised (SIR-R1)

The Statistical Information on Recidivism—Revised (SIR-R1) is an updated version of an instrument originally developed and reported on in the early 1980s (Nuffield, 1982). The Recidivism Prediction Score or General Statistical Information on Recidivism, as it was previously known, was developed to apply statistical information to the parole board release-decision-making process in Canada. Recidivism, both then and now, was defined to be rearrest for an indictable offense during the 3 years following release from prison. The SIR-R1 is still currently scored on offenders within the federal correctional system in Canada. Fifteen risk items were identified (see Table 3.9), the majority of which can be scored from an offender's criminal history (rap sheet). These items were weighted according to the deviation

TABLE 3.9. Items of the SIR-R1

- Current offense
- Age at admission
- Previous incarceration
- Revocation or forfeiture
- Act of escape
- Security classification
- Age at first adult conviction
- Previous convictions for assault
- Marital status at most recent admission
- Interval at risk since last offense
- Number of dependents at most recent admission
- Current total aggregate sentence
- Previous convictions for sex offenses
- Previous convictions for breaking and entering
- Employment status at arrest

from the base rate. To make matters a bit more confusing, it was deviation from success rate rather than failure rate that has resulted in risk categories that are communicated positively (i.e., two out of every three offenders will not commit an indictable offense after release; see Table 3.10). Scores can therefore range from –30 to +27, and these scores have been reduced to five "probability bins" in similar fashion to the LSI-R and the VRAG.

An early peer-reviewed study by Wormith and Goldstone (1984) showed the SIR-R1 to be well associated with general criminal recidivism ($r = .39$). Our research (Mills & Kroner, 2006a) found that in instances in which different assessment instruments disagreed, the SIR-R1 was the most consistently accurate instrument in the prediction of violent recidivism. A list of relevant studies using the SIR-R1 are found in Table 3.11.

The SIR-R1 falls within the public domain and its description and scoring procedures are described in the Commissioner's Directive CD705-6 (see *www.csc-scc.gc.ca/text/plcy/cdshtm/705-6-cd-eng.shtml#_Statitistical*). The 15 items to be rated are as follows: current offense, age at admission, previous incarceration, revocation or forfeiture, act of escape, security classification, age at first adult conviction, previous convictions for assault, marital status at most recent admission, interval at risk since last offense, number of dependents at most recent admission, current total aggregate sentence, previous convictions for sex offenses, previous convictions for breaking and entering, and employment status at arrest.

INSTRUMENTS DEVELOPED TO PREDICT SEXUAL VIOLENCE

As with other risk appraisal instruments, instruments designed to predict sexual and violent recidivism among sex offenders do not consistently differ in the prediction of recidivism. Some studies may show one to be more accurate in absolute terms than another, but not necessarily significantly different to a statistically meaningful degree. In a comparison of nine risk assessment instruments developed to predict sexual recidivism Raymond Knight and David Thornton (2007) concluded that there were not meaningful and consistent differences between the accuracy of the instruments.

TABLE 3.10. Success Rates Based on SIR-R1 Scores

+6 to +27	4 out of every 5 offenders will not commit an indictable offense after release
+1 to +5	2 out of every 3 offenders will not commit an indictable offense after release
–4 to 0	1 out of every 2 offenders will not commit an indictable offense after release
–8 to –5	2 out of every 5 offenders will not commit an indictable offense after release
–30 to –9	1 out of every 3 offenders will not commit an indictable offense after release

TABLE 3.11. Outcomes for Studies Using the SIR

Study	Sample description				Criterion and follow-up	Outcome
	Participants	Sex	Jurisdiction	Race		
Wormith & Goldstone (1984)	Correctional	Male	Canada	Predominantly white	Retrospective, not reported	Any recidivism $r = .39$
Bonta, Harman, Hann, & Cormier (1996)	Correctional	Male	Canada	Predominantly white	Retrospective, 3 years	Any recidivism $r = .42$
Mills, Loza, & Kroner (2003)	Correctional	Male	Canada	Predominantly white	Predictive, not reported	General reoffense $r = .39$; Violent reoffense $r = .29$
Kroner & Loza (2001)	Correctional	Male	Canada	Predominantly white	Predictive, 20 months	Violent recidivism AUC = .74
Mills, Kroner, & Hemmati (2004)	Correctional	Male	Canada	Predominantly white	Predictive, 2 years	General reoffense AUC = .78; violent reoffense AUC = .79
Mills & Kroner (2006a)	Correctional	Male	Canada	Predominantly white	Predictive, 3 years	general reoffense $r = .38$; violent reoffense $r = .30$

88

Jan Looman and Jeff Abracen (2010) did show that a number of risk measures (Rapid Risk Assessment for Sex Offense Recidivism [RRASOR], Static-99) were more accurate when used with rapists but not with child molesters in a sample of high-risk sex offenders. This was not the case, however, in an earlier study that showed the same instruments to be equally accurate for the two different types of sexual offenders (Sjostedt & Langstrom, 2001). Still another study showed the Static-99 to be consistently accurate among sex offender types whereas the RRASOR was most accurate for incest offenders (Bartosh, Garby, Lewis, & Gray, 2003). These findings should not be taken as evidence regarding the inconsistency or inaccuracy of the instruments. Each sample is unique and in most cases methodology differs, which can result in differences in scoring. These differences are not unexpected, particularly in retrospective designs.

Researchers very seldom examine the individual items of risk instruments to determine if the risk factor itself is effective in identifying recidivists. We consider this to be an all-too-frequent oversight. Inclusion of how individual variables perform would be helpful in determining the variables that replicate as effective risk factors across many samples. One example of this is a cross-validation study of the Static-99 and RRASOR to a Swedish sample of correctional sex offenders. An item analysis showed that three of the 10 variables that comprise the Static-99 did not distinguish recidivists from nonrecidivists. This does not mean that the instrument is not valid, rather it may inform us, in conjunction with other studies, on what variables are potentially weaker predictors. This may point to eventual exclusion of the variable or it may mean a recalibration for scoring. Unfortunately, not enough studies report these types of findings.

Rapid Risk Assessment for Sex Offense Recidivism

The RRASOR (Hanson, 1997) is a brief actuarial risk assessment instrument developed by Karl Hanson based on the results of his meta-analysis of the predictors of sexual offender recidivism (Hanson & Bussiere, 1998). Initially, Hanson chose the predictors from the meta-analysis that had an average correlation effect size of 0.10 or greater with the outcome of sexual reoffense. You will recall that we covered this meta-analysis in more detail in Chapter 2. The initial items to choose from included having a prior sex offense, victim was a stranger, any prior offenses, being of young age, having never been married, having nonrelated victims, and having any male victims. These seven variables were analyzed with data from six different studies totaling over 2,000 offenders. Four items were identified as the best combination to most accurately predict the outcome of sexual recidivism: prior sex offenses, age at release, victim gender, and relationship to the victim. These four items were called the RRASOR and were cross-validated on a seventh sample of offenders, producing an AUC of .67 which was comparable to the average AUC = .71 of the samples on which the RRASOR was developed. Recidivism estimates based on the RRASOR score are reported in Table 3.12.

The RRASOR has the advantage of being very quick in identifying high-risk offenders. The RRASOR scores have been associated with recidivism over time; however, with the advent of the Static-99, which is more comprehensive, generally more accurate, and more psychometrically sound, the RRASOR would not be the best choice for a comprehensive assessment for sexual recidivism in our opinion. That said, the RRASOR may be an effective initial classification tool to determine the general level of risk in consultation or screening scenarios where a full assessment has not commenced. Studies reporting the predictive accuracy of the RRASOR are listed in Table 3.13.

Static-99

The Static-99 was originally developed by Karl Hanson and David Thornton (2000) following an analysis that showed that the combined instruments of the RRASOR (Hanson, 1997) and the Structured Anchored Clinical Judgment (SACJ-Min; Grubin, 1998) were better predictors of sexual reoffense outcome than either instrument alone. The items from each of these scales were combined to create the 10-item Static-99 (see Table 3.14). Because of the public policy importance of managing sex offenders and the accuracy and simplicity of scoring the Static-99, it has become arguably the most widely used actuarial instrument in the world to assess violence and the most studied (Hanson & Morton-Bourgon, 2007). However, with its wide use has come increased scrutiny through multiple court challenges that have served to clarify with increased specificity how each of the 10 items are to be scored. As a result, the most recent edition of the Static-99 Coding

TABLE 3.12. RRASOR Sexual Recidivism Estimates

RRASOR Score	5 years	10 years	Doren (2004)
0	4.4%	6.5%	3.8%
1	7.6%	11.2%	9.3%
2	14.2%	21.1%	11.5%
3	24.8%	36.9%	27.7%
4	32.7%	48.6%	33.8%
5	49.8%	73.1%	47.25%

Note. Five- and 10-year percentages are from Hanson (1997). Doren (2004a) aggregated 10 independent studies and compared them with the Hanson (1997) 5-year rates.

TABLE 3.13. Outcomes for Studies Using the RRASOR

Study	Sample description				Criterion and follow-up	Outcome
	Participants	Sex	Jurisdiction	Race		
Hanson & Thorton (2000)	Sex offenders	Male	Multinational	Not reported	Retrospective, up to 15 years	Sexual offense AUC = .68
Barbaree, Seto, Langton, & Peacock (2001)	Correctional sex offenders	Male	Canada	Mixed	Retrospective, 4.5 years	Violent offense AUC = .65; sexual offense AUC = .77
Sjostedt & Langstrom (2001)	Correctional sex offenders	Male	Sweden	Predominantly white	Retrospective, 3.7 years	Sexual offense AUC = .72; violent offense AUC = .63
Bartosh, Garby, Lewis, & Gray (2003)	Correctional sex offenders	Male	United States	Mixed	Retrospective, 5 years	Sexual offense AUC = .63
Harris et al. (2003)	1. Forensic inpatients 2. Correctional psychiatric	Male Male	Canada Canada	Mixed Mixed	Predictive, 3 years Predictive, 3 years	Sexual offenses AUC = .63 Sexual offenses AUC = .61
	3. Correctional psychiatric	Male	Canada	Mixed	Predictive, 3 years	Sexual offenses AUC = .52
Langton et al. (2007)	Sexual offenders	Male	Canada	Not reported	Retrospective, 3 years	Sexual reoffending AUC = .77
Knight & Thornton (2007)	Correctional sex offenders	Male	United States	Predominantly white	Retrospective, fixed 3, 10, & 15 years	Sexual re-offending 3-year AUC = .67; 10-year AUC = .68
Looman & Abracen (2010)	Sex offenders in forensic hospital	Male	Canada	Not reported	Retrospective, 7 years	Sexual offense AUC = .62; violent and sexual offenses AUC = .55

TABLE 3.14. Items of the Static-99

* Age
* Ever lived with an intimate partner for at least 2 years
* Any convictions among index offenses nonsexual violence
* Any convictions for prior nonsexual violence
* Prior sex offenses
* Prior sentencing dates (excluding index)
* Any convictions for noncontact sex offenses
* Any unrelated victims
* Any stranger victims
* Any male victims

Rules (Harris, Phenix, Hanson, & Thornton, 2003) is 80 pages with future additions pending.

The 10 items of the Static-99 include age, ever lived with an intimate partner for 2 years, conviction for a nonsexual violent offense at the same time as the conviction for the current sex offense, conviction for a prior nonsexual violent offense, convictions for prior sex offenses, four or more prior sentencing dates, convictions for noncontact sex offenses, any unrelated victims, any stranger victims, and any male victims. Scores on the Static-99 can range from 0 to 12; however, the sample size for the groups of offenders scoring above 6 becomes smaller and therefore provides less reliable information. Interpretation of scores typically include the score bins from 0, 1, 2, 3, 4, 5, and 6+. The length of follow-up also permits the inclusion of recidivism rates over time and the scoring guide includes periods of 5, 10, and 15 years with recidivism rates tending to increase linearly across both score and time periods (see Table 3.15).

The Static-99 has been cross-validated numerous times. A recent meta-analysis identified 42 research studies that employed the instrument to study sexual reoffense in a combined sample exceeding 13,000 offenders (Hanson & Morton-Bourgon, 2007). Hanson (2006) reported on over 3,400 sexual offenders and showed that the Static-99 was effective at identifying recidivists across age groups, even among those over the age of 60 years. Given that a reduction in recidivism has been shown to be associated with increased age, Hanson (2006) recalculated risk probabilities associated with scores on the Static-99 for various age groups over a 5-year period. Those rates are included here as an adjunct to the rates that are reported in the original Static-99 study (Table 3.16).

The authors of the Static-99 recommend that individuals who choose

TABLE 3.15. Sexual Recidivism Rates for the Static-99 Scores

	Years postrelease		
Static-99 score	5 years	10 years	15 years
0	5%	11%	13%
1	6%	7%	7%
2	9%	13%	16%
3	12%	14%	19%
4	26%	31%	36%
5	33%	38%	40%
6+	39%	45%	52%

Note. Data from Hanson and Thornton (2000).

to use the instrument should receive training in the scoring of the instrument. Current information on the Static-99 can be found on the website *www.static99.org*. Recidivism rates as current as October 2008 are available at this website for both 5- and 10-year follow-up periods.

Static-2002

The Static-99 has been revised as the Static-2002 (Hanson & Thornton, 2003), which is currently being cross-validated as more studies employ the instrument (Langton, Barbaree, Hansen, Harkins, & Peacock, 2007). Some studies have found a relatively dramatic improvement in the Static-2002 over the Static-99 in predictive accuracy (Looman & Abracen, 2010), while other studies have found it to be statistically the same with the Static-99 being marginally more accurate (Knight & Thornton, 2007; Langton, Barbaree, Seto, et al., 2007).

TABLE 3.16. Probability of Sexual Recidivism by Static-99 Score and Offender Age

		Age at Release				
Risk category	Score	18–24.9	25–39.9	40–40.9	50–59.9	60+
Low	0–1	5.8	6.7%	5.5%	2.5%	0.0%
Moderate–low	2–3	7.6%	11.7%	6.7%	4.3%	3.0%
Moderate–high	4–5	24.6%	24.3%	13.8%	19.4%	4.8%
High	6–12	35.5%	37.5%	25.7%	24.3%	9.1%

Note. Data from Hanson (2006).

However, at the present time the Static-99 is the most rigorously studied instrument and is the only version reported here. It is possible that in the future, with additional empirical support, the Static-2002 may replace the Static-99. A relevant list of studies using the Static-99 is reported in Table 3.17.

Stable-2007 and Acute-2007

The Stable-2007 and the Acute-2007 were developed out of research conducted by Karl Hanson and Andrew Harris in Canada. Their initial work identified dynamic or changeable risk variables associated with sexual reoffending (Hanson & Harris, 2000). From this initial study these researchers developed the Sex Offender Need Assessment Rating (SONAR), which was validated based upon a retrospective study that compared sex offender recidivists with sex offender nonrecidivists (Hanson & Harris, 2001). The resulting dynamic risk factors were initially referred to as the Stable-2007 and the Acute-2000 and with some revisions are called the Stable-2007 and the Acute-2007. These scales in conjunction with the Static-99 are consistent with a dynamic–actuarial approach to risk assessment and in our opinion hold much promise for the future in sex offender risk. The Dynamic Supervision Project is a research endeavor that prospectively applied the Static-99, the Stable-2007, and the Acute-2007 across all jurisdictions in Canada as well as in Iowa and Alaska in the United States. The initial findings reported on nearly 1,000 offenders who were tracked and reassessed by their parole and probation officers for an average of 41 months. The reliability assessment showed excellent performance with the Static-99 but less so for the Stable and the Acute. The purpose of this research project was to demonstrate the utility of dynamic variables in the assessment and management of risk.

The results of the study were very encouraging. All predictors were moderately associated with the two sexual offense outcomes (see Table 3.18): sexual crime recidivism (any sexual crime including noncontact and consenting such as prostitution) and any sexual recidivism (including sexual crime recidivism as well as breaches for violations related to sexual offending). In addition, the Acute-2007, as measured within the 45 days prior to the reoffense, added to the Static-99/Stable-2007 risk rating in predicting sexual reoffending. From an applied perspective, the combination of the Static-99, the Stable-2007, and the Acute-2007 theoretically permits some adjustment to the offender's overall risk characterization by modifying somewhat the individual's original static risk classification and it is consistent with a *dynamic–actuarial* risk assessment approach. However, in practice, the changes in the dynamic variables did not improve predictive accuracy. Nonetheless, this combination of static and dynamic variables

TABLE 3.17. Outcomes for Studies Using the Static-99

Study	Sample description				Criterion and follow-up	Outcome
	Participants	Sex	Jurisdiction	Race		
Hanson & Thorton (2000)[a]	Sex offenders	Male	Multinational	Not reported	Retrospective, up to 15 years	Sexual offense AUC = .71
Barbaree, Seto, Langton, & Peacock (2001)	Correctional sex offenders	Male	Canada	Mixed	Retrospective, 4.5 years	Violent offense AUC = .70; sexual offense AUC = .70
Sjostedt & Langstrom (2001)	Correctional sex offenders	Male	Sweden	Predominantly white	Retrospective, 3.7 years	Sexual offense AUC = .76; violent offense AUC = .74
Bartosh, Garby, Lewis, & Gray (2003)	Correctional sex offenders	Male	United States	Mixed	Retrospective, 5 years	Sexual offense AUC = .64
Harris, Rice et al. (2003)	1. Forensic inpatients 2. Correctional psychiatric	Male Male	Canada Canada	Mixed Mixed	Predictive, 3 years Predictive, 3 years	Sexual offenses AUC = .67 Sexual offenses AUC = .63
	3. Correctional psychiatric	Male	Canada	Mixed	Predictive, 3 years	Sexual offenses AUC = .54
de Vodel, de Ruiter, van Beek, & Mead (2004)	Forensic hospital sex offenders	Male	Netherlands	Not reported	Retrospective, 11.5 years	Sexual offense AUC = .71; violent offense AUC = .54
Stadtland et al. (2005)	Correctional offenders	Male	Germany	Not reported	Retrospective, 9 years	Sexual offenses AUC = .66; violent offenses AUC = .71

(continued)

TABLE 3.17. (continued)

Study	Participants	Sample description Sex	Jurisdiction	Race	Criterion and follow-up	Outcome
Ducro & Pham (2006)	Hospitalized sex offenders	Male	Belgium	Not reported	Retrospective, 4.2 years	Sexual Offense AUC = .66; nonsexual violence AUC = .68
Hanson (2006)	Mixed	Male	Multinational	Mixed	Mixed	Sexual recidivism AUC = .70
Langton, Barbaree, Seto, et al. (2007)	Sexual offenders	Made	Canada	Not reported	Retrospective, 3 years	Sexual reoffending AUC = .75
Allan, Grace, Rutherford, & Hudson (2007)	Child molesters	Male	New Zealand	Predominantly white	Retrospective, 5.8 years	Sexual offense AUC = .72
Knight & Thornton (2007)	Correctional sex offenders	Male	United States	Predominantly white	Retrospective, fixed 3, 10, & 15 years	Sexual reoffending 3-year AUC = .71; 10-year AUC = .68
Endrass, Urbaniok, Held, Vetter, & Rossegger (2008)	Forensic	Male	Switzerland	Not reported	Retrospective, 5 years	Sexual reoffense AUC = .76 (based on risk categories)
Kingston, Yates, Firestone, Babchishin, & Bradford (2008)	Sex offenders; Psychiatric hospital outpatients	Male	Canada	Not reported	Retrospective, 11.4 years	Sexual offense AUC = .76 Violent and sexual offense AUC = .70
Looman & Abracen (2010)	Sex offenders in forensic hospital	Male	Canada	Not reported	Retrospective, 7 years	Sexual offense AUC = .59; violent and sexual offense AUC = .58

[a]Construction sample.

96

TABLE 3.18. AUCs and Reoffending from the Dynamic Supervision Project

Measure	Sexual crime	Any sexual recidivism
Static-99	.74	.69
Stable-2007	.67	.69
Acute-2007	.74	.65

Note. Data from Hanson, Harris, Scott, and Helmus (2007).

provides a comprehensive assessment of sex offender risk as well as identifies targets for intervention and management. The procedure for scoring these instruments and applying them to sex offender risk assessment is fairly complex and not for the uninitiated. The developers strongly recommend appropriate training before undertaking risk assessment with these instruments, but the results are good news for the advancement of sex offender risk assessment.

Risk Matrix 2000

The Risk Matrix 2000 (RM2000; Thornton, 2005; Thornton et al., 2003) was developed to predict both sexual and violent reoffending among sex offenders. The RM2000 evolved from a previous instrument, the Structured Anchored Clinical Judgment. The RM2000 comprises three scales: the RM2000/S, which predicts sexual recidivism, the RM2000/V, which predicts nonsexual violence, and the RM2000/C, which combines the first two scales to predict both sexual and other types of violence. Scoring the RM2000/S is done in two steps. In the first step, age, sexual crimes, and criminal offenses are awarded points so that the resulting total varies from 0 to 6 points. The points are then categorized into one of four descriptive classifications: low (0 points), medium (1–2 points), high (3–4 points), and very high (5–6 points). In the second step the presence or absence of four aggravating factors is determined: male victim of sex offense, stranger victim of sex offense, single—never married, and noncontact sex offense. The original descriptive categories above are then changed according to three rules: no change if 0 or 1 aggravating factors are present, increase the risk category one level if 2 or 3 aggravating factors are present, and increase the risk category two levels if all four aggravating factors are present.

Scoring the RM2000/V is much simpler. Three risk factors have been identified. These include age, violent offenses, and burglary. Points are awarded on the basis of these three risk factors, which result in the following risk categorization: low (0–1 point), medium (2–3 points), high (4 to 5 points), and very high (6+ points). The combined risk scale results from adding the RM2000/S and RM2000/V after applying values of low risk = 0, medium risk = 1, high risk = 2, and very high risk = 3. The resulting scale of 0 to 6 points is classified as follows: low (0 points), medium (1–2 points), high (3–4) points, and very high (5–6 points). The items for the RM2000 are listed in Table 3.19.

Craig et al. (2006) compared the RM2000 with the Static-99 in a sample that combined sexual offenders with violent offenders and found only marginal predictive accuracy for both instruments; this was attributed to combining offender types in the same sample. Drew Kingston and colleagues (Kingston, Yates, Firestone, Babchishin, & Bradford, 2008) examined the RM2000 in a retrospective study of sex offenders in an outpatient treatment program. They found the RM2000 to be moderately to strongly related to the Static-99 and the SORAG. However, the predictive accuracy of the Static-99 and the SORAG exceeded that of the RM2000 over the average follow-up time of 11 years. The risk categories were not stable in terms of recidivism percentages when compared with the RM2000 sample of origin. A list of relevant outcome studies utilizing the RM2000 is found in Table 3.20.

Sexual Violence Risk-20

The Sexual Violence Risk-20 (SVR-20) is an SPJ instrument much like the HCR-20 in that it has identified 20 risk factors (see Table 3.21) that broadly fall within the domains of psychosocial adjustment, sexual offending, and

TABLE 3.19. Items of the RM2000

RM2000—Sex

• Number of sentencing appearances for sex offense

• Number of sentencing appearance for any criminal offense

• Age upon release

• Male victim of a sexual offense

• Stranger victim of a sexual offense

• Single, never married

• Noncontact sex offense

RM2000—Violence

• Age

• Violent offenses

• Burglary

TABLE 3.20. Outcomes for Studies Using the RM2000

Study	Sample description				Criterion and follow-up	Outcome
	Participants	Sex	Jurisdiction	Race		
Craig, Beech, & Browne (2006)	Sex offenders	Male	United Kingdom	Not reported	Retrospective, 8 years	Sexual offense AUC = .59
Knight & Thornton (2007)	Correctional Sex offenders	Male	United States	Predominantly white	Retrospective, fixed 3, 10, & 15 years	Sexual reoffending 3-year AUC = .67, 10-year AUC = .64
Kingston, Yates, Firestone, Babchishin, & Bradford (2008)	Sex Offenders Psychiatric hospital outpatients	Male	Canada	Not reported	Retrospective, 11.4 years	Sexual offense AUC = .65 Violent and sexual offense AUC = .64
Looman & Abracen (2010)	Sex offenders in forensic hospital	Male	Canada	Not reported	Retrospective, 7 years	Sexual offense AUC = .66; violent and sexual offense AUC = .71

TABLE 3.21. Items of the SVR-20

Part A: Psychosocial adjustment
1. Sexual deviation
2. Victim of child abuse
3. Psychopathy
4. Major mental illness
5. Substance abuse problems
6. Suicidal/homicidal ideation
7. Relationship problems
8. Employment problems
9. Past nonsexual violence
10. Past nonviolent offending
11. Past supervision failures
Part B: Sex offenses
12. High-density sexual offending
13. Multiple sex offense type
14. Physical harm to victim
15. Uses weapons or threats of death
16. Escalation in frequency or severity
17. Extreme minimization or denial
18. Attitudes that support sex offending
Part C: Future plans
19. Lacks realistic plans
20. Negative attitude toward intervention

future plans. One of the first published investigations into the validity of the SVR-20 found that 11 of the 20 risk factors did not correlate significantly with sexual recidivism (Dempster & Hart, 2002). These included some factors such as denial of sex offenses that have been shown in meta-analyses not to be related to sexual reoffending but also others such as sexual deviation that have been considered central to sexual recidivism. Despite the poor performance of individual items, the overall instrument has been shown to be associated with sexual reoffending in a number of studies (see Table 3.22). Validity of the SVR-20 has been found in different countries, though the studies have been retrospective in design. Predictive accuracy has var-

TABLE 3.22. Outcomes for Studies Using the SVR-20

Study	Sample description			Criterion and follow-up	Outcome
	Participants	Sex	Jurisdiction	Race		

Study	Participants	Sex	Jurisdiction	Race	Criterion and follow-up	Outcome
Sjostdet & Langstrom (2002)	Forensic hospital sex offenders	Male	Sweden	Not reported	Retrospective, 6 years	Sexual violence AUC = .49
de Vogel, de Ruiter, van Beek, & Mead (2004)	Forensic hospital sex offenders	Male	Netherlands	Not reported	Retrospective, 11.5 years	Sexual offense AUC = .80, Violent offense AUC = .66
Craig, Beech, & Browne (2006)	Sex offenders	Males	United Kingdom	Not reported	Retrospective, 10 years	Sexual offense AUC = .51
Stadtland et al. (2005)	Correctional offenders	Male	Germany	Not reported	Retrospective, 9 years	Sexual offenses AUC = .68, Violent offenses AUC = .68
Knight & Thornton (2007)	Correctional sex offenders	Male	United States	Predominantly white	Retrospective, fixed 3, 10, & 15 years	Sexual reoffending 3-year AUC = .66; 10-year AUC = .68

ied from chance levels in Sweden and the United Kingdom to very good in the Netherlands. The SVR-20 is commercially available through the Mental Health, Law, and Policy Institute of Simon Fraser University (*www.sfu.ca/ mhlpi/publications.htm*) or Psychological Assessment Resources, Inc.

Violence Risk Scale: Sex Offender Version

Mark Olver and colleagues developed and published the Violence Risk Scale: Sex Offender Version (VRS-SO) based on a retrospective study that examined both static and potentially dynamic variables of 321 male federal offenders who participated in a high-intensity sex offender treatment program (Olver et al., 2007). This scale falls into the category of dynamic–actuarial risk assessment and we believe is one that has future potential. Similar to the VRS, the VRS-SO has seven static items and 17 dynamic items which are rated on a 4-point 0–3 Likert-type scale. For each of the 17 dynamic items the five stages of change have been operationalized (see the transtheoretical model of change of Prochaska, DiClemente, & Norcross, 1992) in order to measure treatment change on the specific dynamic item.

A factor analysis of the dynamic items yielded three factors that represented sexual deviance, criminality, and treatment responsivity. The VRS-SO static measure was correlated with the Static-99. The average follow-up time was 10 years and the predictive accuracy of the VRS-SO was consistent with other measures of sexual offender recidivism: VRS-SO Static AUC = .74, VRS-SO Dynamic AUC = .66, Static-99 AUC = .63. An important finding in this study was that change due to treatment was related to a change in risk, specifically, that positive change was related to decreased sexual recidivism. This finding is very encouraging for the advancement of risk assessment in general and sex offender risk assessment specifically as it represents what we have referred to as the *dynamic–actuarial* assessment of risk. With prospective replication comes the hope that changes in risk resulting from treatment may actually be quantified statistically, resulting in greater accuracy as well as giving the clients credit for the efforts made to address their deviant behavior.

INSTRUMENTS DEVELOPED
TO PREDICT SPOUSAL VIOLENCE

Spousal Assault Risk Assessment Guide

The scoring guide to the original Spousal Assault Risk Assessment Guide (SARA) was first released in 1994, revised in 1995, and then made commercially available in 1999 (Kropp, Hart, Webster, & Eaves, 1994, 1995, 1999). The SARA comprises 20 items that fall within four domains (see

Table 3.23). The first domain is *general criminal history*, which is measured by items that document past assault of family members, past assault of strangers or acquaintances, and past violations of conditional release. *Psychosocial adjustment* is the second domain, measured by the items of relationship problems, employment problems, victim or witness of family violence when a child, substance abuse/dependence, recent suicidal or homicidal thoughts, recent psychotic or manic symptoms, and personality disorder with anger, impulsivity, or behavioral instability. These first two domains combine to create what Kropp and Hart (2000) refer to as "general violence risk factors." *Spousal assault history* is the third domain, measured by the items of past physical assault, prior sexual assault/sexual jealousy, prior use of threats or weapons, recent escalation in frequency or severity of assault, past violation of no-contact orders, extreme minimization or denial of spousal assault, and attitudes that support spousal assault. The last and fourth domain pertains to the *most recent offense*. The three items relevant to this domain are severe and/or sexual assault, use of weapons and/or cred-

TABLE 3.23. Items of the SARA

- Prior assault of family members
- Prior assault of strangers or acquaintances
- Prior violation of conditional release
- Recent relationship problems
- Recent employment problems
- Victim of and/or witness to family violence in youth
- Recent substance abuse
- Recent suicidal or homicidal thoughts
- Recent psychotic or manic symptoms
- Personality disorder
- Prior assault of spouse
- Prior sexual assault or sexual jealousy of spouse
- Past use of weapons or threats of death toward spouse
- Past violation of no-contact orders
- Minimization or denial of spouse abuse
- Attitudes that condone spouse abuse
- Severe and/or sexual assault in recent offense
- Use of weapons or threats of death in recent offense
- Violation of no-contact order in recent offense

ible threats of death, and violation of no-contact order. These latter two domains combine to create what are referred to as "spousal violence risk factors." Each of these items are scored from 0 (not present) to 2 (present) and the resulting score ranges from 0 to 40. In addition to the score, the number of risk factors identified as present is also tabulated. The authors have provided tables and suggested cutoffs between low-to-moderate and moderate-to-high ranges. The determination of the ultimate risk rating is left to the discretion of the rater.

Concurrent validity of the SARA was reported by Kropp and Hart (2000). Their study showed that the SARA general violence risk factors were correlated with other risk scales developed to predict both general and violent reoffending. Also, in a comparison of 50 nonrecidivists with 52 spouse assault recidivists, the latter group scored higher on the aggregate score of the SARA spousal assault risk factors and there was a trend in the same direction for the general violence risk factors.

An international cross-validation effort in Sweden reported a moderate level of predictive accuracy (Grann & Wedin, 2002). The SARA was appropriately correlated with other instruments that had been retrospectively scored on this sample such as the PCL-R and the VRAG. After a 5-year average follow-up time and a recidivism rate of 28%, the predictive accuracy of the SARA for spousal assault recidivism was moderate (AUC = .65). These authors identified the items of past violation of conditional release; personality disorder with anger, impulsivity; or behavioral instability, and extreme minimization as having particular importance in distinguishing between recidivists and nonrecidivists. The mean SARA score was 20 points, which would suggest that this sample was a much higher risk than the original sample on which the scale was developed.

In their construction of the Ontario Domestic Assault Risk Assessment, Hilton et al. (2004) scored the SARA without all the information that the SARA authors required. On one sample of approximately 320 cases the SARA had an AUC of .64 with future spousal assault. On a second smaller sample of 100 spouse abusers the SARA did not predict future spouse abuse (AUC = .54). Elsewhere, the SARA was more accurate than the Domestic Violence Screening Instrument in a large sample of spouse abusers (Williams & Houghton, 2004). A list of relevant studies are reported in Table 3.24.

The SARA is commercially available through Multi-Health Systems, Inc. (www.mhs.com).

Ontario Domestic Assault Risk Assessment and Domestic Violence Risk Appraisal Guide

In 2004, Zoe Hilton and colleagues published their findings on the development and validation of the Ontario Domestic Assault Risk Assessment

TABLE 3.24. Outcomes for Studies Using the SARA

| | Sample description | | | | Criterion and | |
Study	Participants	Sex	Jurisdiction	Race	follow-up	Outcome
Grann & Wedin (2002)	Forensic patients	Male	Sweden	Not reported	Retrospective, 5 years	Spousal assault Part 1 AUC = .59, Part 2 AUC = .62; total score AUC = .65
Williams & Houghton (2004)	Spouse assaulters	Male	United States	Not reported	Predictive, 18 months	Spousal assault AUC = .65
Hilton et al. (2004)	Arrestees for spousal assault	Male	Canada	Not reported	Retrospective, 51 months	Spousal assault AUC = .64 and AUC = .54[a]
Hilton, Harris, Rice, Houghton, & Eke, (2008)	Spouse assaulters	Male	Canada	Not reported	Retrospective, 5 years	Spousal assault AUC = .59

[a]Authors reported that not all information was available to code the SARA according to the manual.

(ODARA; Hilton et al., 2004). The ODARA's development mirrored in many ways the development of the VRAG and the SORAG. These researchers reviewed the detailed police reports of 589 incidents involving a man who physically assaulted his current or former common-law partner or wife. Thirty-eight risk factors were identified. These included the Domestic Violence Supplementary Report (DVSR; Ontario Ministry of the Solicitor General, 2000) and in approximately half of the cases there was sufficient information to score the Danger Assessment (DA; Campbell, 1986) and the Spousal Assault Risk Assessment (SARA; Kropp et al., 1999). Interestingly, the DVSR, the DA, and the SARA were equivalent with certain single risk factors such as the perpetrator's substance abuse score, prior domestic incidents, and prior correctional sentence in his relationship with spouse assault recidivism. The items selected for the ODARA are found in Table 3.25. The base rate in this construction sample was 30% over a 51-month time frame. The ODARA's point-biserial correlation with spouse assault was strong ($r = .43$), as was its ROC (AUC = .77). It is to be expected that indices of relationship and accuracy will almost certainly be best on the sample in

TABLE 3.25. Items of the ODARA

- Prior domestic incident
- Prior nondomestic incident
- Prior correctional sentence
- Conditional release failure
- Threat to harm or kill at recent incident
- Confinement during recent incident
- Victim concern
- More than one child
- Victim has biological child from a previous partner
- Violence against others
- Substance abuse
- Assault on victim when pregnant
- Barriers to victim support

which the instrument was developed because of the capitalization on variance unique to the sample.

Hilton and colleagues cross-validated the ODARA on 100 spouse assaulters. The base rate in this sample was slightly lower at 26%. As expected, the correlation and ROC with recidivism was reduced from the construction sample but still quite robust at $r = .36$ and AUC = .72. The ODARA also correlated with other measures of spouse abuse such as the DA ($r = .43$), the SARA ($r = .60$), and the DVSR ($r = .53$). Of note, none of these latter assessment instruments were significantly accurate in their prediction of recidivism in the validation sample. Interrater reliability of the ODARA was very good for both research assistants (ICC = .90) and police officers (ICC = .95). Hilton and Harris (2009) cross-validated the ODARA on a sample with a lower base rate and found the predictive accuracy to be in the moderate range (AUC = .67). A list of relevant studies is reported in Table 3.26.

In a recent revision Zoe Hilton and colleagues revisited the ODARA and added the score of the PCL-R to create a new instrument that they have called the Domestic Violence Risk Appraisal Guide (DVRAG; Hilton, Harris, et al., 2008). Improvements in predictive accuracy were found and replicated by adding the PCL-R. Scores of the DVRAG are weighted in a similar manner as the VRAG and the SORAG and scores are divided into one of seven predictive bins each with an associated recidivism rate. Unfortunately, in the addition of psychopathy (PCL-R) to the DVRAG, the authors did not

TABLE 3.26. Outcomes for Studies Using the ODARA

| | Sample description | | | | | |
Study	Participants	Sex	Jurisdiction	Race	Criterion and follow-up	Outcome
Hilton et al. (2004)	Arrestees for spousal assault	Male	Canada	Not reported	Retrospective, 51 months	Spousal assault AUC = .72
Hilton & Harris (2009)	Arrestees for spousal assault	Male	Canada	Not reported	Retrospective, 5 years	Spousal assault AUC = .67
Hilton, Harris, Rice, Houghton, & Eke (2008)	Spouse assaulters	Male	Canada	Not reported	Retrospective, 5 years	Spousal assault AUC = .65

report the relative contribution of the two underlying factors or the four facets. As you will recall from the previous discussion on psychopathy it seems that it is the criminal lifestyle component that is most strongly related to crime and violence. Additionally, it would appear that the actual psychopath versus nonpsychopath distinction is not the issue within the context of the DVRAG as evidenced by the mean PCL-R scores and standard deviations. The mean PCL-R score in the validation sample was 8.4, with a standard deviation of 6.7. This means that approximately 80% of the spouse abuse sample had scores below that of the average violent criminal.

In a recent book published by Hilton, Harris, and Rice (2009) the authors have combined the ODARA and the DVRAG into a system for assessing domestic violence risk. The ODARA is presented as a risk appraisal instrument for frontline personnel (police, victim counselors, etc.) who require a relatively quick and reliable index of risk. The DVRAG is presented as a risk appraisal instrument for use by forensic professionals who have access to more information and in instances where a more formal evaluation is necessary. Scoring procedures for both instruments is provided in the Hilton, Harris, and Rice (2009) publication.

CHAPTER 4

■　■　■

ISSUES IN RISK ASSESSMENT

As recently as 15 years ago, the development of a list of violence risk appraisal instruments would have been a brief exercise. There simply were not enough published instruments to develop a multiple-step guideline for choosing an instrument. During such times (mostly during the 1980s and early 1990s) a basic knowledge of an instrument's strengths and weaknesses, validity, and reliability could suffice as criteria for choosing an instrument and defending your choice during cross-examination. In a more recent review, Otto and Heilbrun (2002) commented that the number of commercially available instruments has increased dramatically. This is supported from our review of the risk appraisal instruments in Chapter 3, where we identified multiple instruments for different outcomes from varied risk assessment perspectives (SPJ, actuarial). This trend has continued and in the current milieu, with many risk appraisal instruments available, further knowledge is required to rationally select one over others. This knowledge should include psychometric knowledge specific to risk assessment as well as the contextual application of the instrument. Correctly applying this knowledge to a specific assessment situation will require careful consideration, as often a risk appraisal instrument will not correspond directly to the legal or referral question (Packer, 2008).

We concur with the recommendation (see Heilbrun et al., 2007) of not answering the ultimate legal question. For example, a clinician would conduct a risk assessment to determine the likelihood of reoffending, but not express an opinion about whether a parole board should release a specific offender. However, the closer an instrument's supporting research is to the referral question, the greater the transparency when communicating the meaning of the associated risk findings. Not only is a risk assessment instrument unlikely to map directly onto the legal or referral question, but rarely will a clinician apply a violence risk appraisal instrument within the same setting as the instrument's sample of development. Given these realities and the development of many new risk appraisal instruments, what criteria should a clinician use to choose an instrument for a particular evaluation?

CHOOSING A RISK APPRAISAL INSTRUMENT

Choosing a risk assessment instrument necessitates knowledge in three areas: the instruments that are available, the basic psychometric properties of those instruments, and the appropriate criteria for deciding on a specific instrument. In order to work through the assumptions and criteria for choosing an instrument, one needs to have a broad and theoretical understanding of behavior, cognitions, and emotions that contribute to violence. Also, one should understand the assessment of these areas and the outcome of violence. With most instruments a well-trained technician can adequately complete and score the results. However, to understand the research well and make a best-practice decision in choosing and applying a risk appraisal instrument, reporting those findings in a meaningful and accurate way, and identifying risk management strategies based on the findings requires much more than simple knowledge on how to complete a risk appraisal instrument correctly.

The Clinician and Answering the Legal Question

In some circumstances within a legal setting the clinician is called upon to answer a question of direct relevance to the court, for example, the determination of competence to stand trial. Competence depends directly upon the individual's mental functioning which the clinician has been called to assess and to render an opinion—determining competence is the task. In instances of violence risk assessment, the task is assessing the likelihood of an individual acting in a violent manner and this is separate from the judgment of the legal issue at hand, which may be suitability for release from a correctional or forensic facility. In this instance the clinical task of assessment is not the legal issue or decision. The risk to society is quantified by the clinician, but the tolerance of risk is the qualitative determination for society's representatives, the court or judicial board. For these reasons in instances of violence risk assessment we encourage clinicians to avoid commenting or rendering an opinion on the ultimate legal decision.

Instruments Available

When considering the instruments available for use there will not be a "perfect" instrument for the risk assessment situation, only a "better" instrument. Even the better instrument may not be the best choice as more research is conducted and more instruments become available. It is wise periodically to revisit the instruments available for selection. An error of omission (i.e., not including an appropriate instrument because you were unaware of its availability) could be embarrassing if you routinely conduct risk assessments and overlook an important advance (Packer, 2008). If risk assessments are a regular activity in your work, plan to review the risk assessment literature every few months. If your assessments are less frequent, then a review at the time of your assessment is in order.

Psychometric Properties

The risk appraisal instruments you choose should be psychometrically sound for your intended purpose and client population. Prior to outlining the guidelines for choosing an instrument it is assumed that basic psychometric properties have been covered in a manual. A manual does not necessarily need to be commercially published, but research on the instrument should be published in peer-reviewed journals to increase the likelihood the instrument meets the *Daubert* criteria (see Chapter 1 for a review of *Daubert* criteria). As the clinician, you are responsible for selecting appropriate instruments, and that requires your knowledge and understanding of both favorable and unfavorable empirical data on the outcome of interest. Although predictive accuracy is a primary concern with violence risk appraisal instruments, predictive validity alone is not sufficient to warrant instrument selection. In fact, given the number of risk assessment instruments with adequate predictive validity, this is less of an issue when choosing between risk appraisal instruments.

Reliability is a key psychometric quality. First, it is an essential psychometric principle for instrument construction and interpretation, and second, the law requires evidence to be reliable. It should be noted that not all types of reliability apply to all risk appraisal instruments. With actuarial instruments comprising static/historical risk factors chosen according to the relation with an outcome, a coefficient alpha is not necessary as it reflects the internal consistency of a construct and a risk appraisal instrument is not a construct. An instrument having interrater reliability is essential (Austin, 2006). Without evidence that the chosen instrument is reliable when the same client is rated by different clinicians the potential for criticism increases. Inter-rater reliabilities must be adequate (we recommend .70 and

---

Instruments as Evidence

The law also requires that scientific evidence be based on reliable methods. Under Rule 702 of the Federal Rules of Evidence, it states, "if scientific, technical, or other specialized knowledge will assist the trier of fact to understand the evidence or to determine a fact in issue, a witness qualified as an expert by knowledge, skill, experience, training, or education may testify thereto in the form of an opinion or otherwise if (1) the testimony is based upon sufficient facts or data, (2) the testimony is the product of reliable principles and methods, and (3) the witness has applied the principles and methods reliably to the facts of the case" (Fed. R. Evid. 702, 2000). Given the combined legal and psychometric requirements, reliability of the instrument of choice is very important.

---

above) or this alone is a reason to discard an instrument from use in risk assessments.

Choosing an Appropriate Risk Appraisal Instrument

You need to consider not only the psychometric soundness of an instrument but also its relevance in a specific risk assessment situation. We list the criteria below according to general importance, although there may be specialized risk situations where the lower criteria may be alternated.

Normative Relevance

The first issue in choosing a risk assessment instrument is how closely your clients' characteristics match a sample from a predictive study. This is an issue of normative relevance. Stated differently, the closer your client is to a normative sample, the more confidence you may have that the risk appraisal instrument is accurately assessing your client. The validity and base rates of individual variables (risk factors) can differ between groups and change over time. Moreover, culture and criminal justice policies change over time. For example, the meaning and use of tattoos are substantially different now than 15 years ago (see Rozycki, Morgan, Murray, & Varghese, in press). If using the Lifestyle Criminality Screening Form (Walters, White, & Denney, 1991), which contains an item for the presence of a tattoo, current norms would need to be kept in mind given the proliferation of tattooing in popular culture. This is not to say that the tattoo variable has lost its predictive power; rather, the meaning and subsequent interpretation of the specific item in relation to other items will likely have changed. Using different gender norms should also be a priority.

Research indicates that the basic predictors are much the same for men and women, but with different outcome measures base rates for women offenders, and the risk factors can interact differently (Dowden & Andrews, 1999). This appears to be the same for other demographic groups, such as ethic minorities. A well-researched risk appraisal instrument can perform well across ethnic groups (LSI-R, Bonta, 1989; HCR-20, Fujii, Tokioka, Lichton, & Hishinuma, 2005), but the specifics contributing to the overall risk level may vary. For example, Fujii et al. (2005) found the HCR-20 to predict equally well among Asian American, European-American, and Native Hawaiian groups. However, impulsivity was more prominent within the Asian American group and relationship instability more prominent within the Native Hawaiian group.

Range of risk may also have to be considered when selecting your risk appraisal instrument. If your general client group is considered high risk, then instruments with a potential ceiling effect (too many individuals fall within the high-risk group according to the instrument) may not be appropriate. For example, with a psychiatric sample, Belfrage et al. (2000) found that the historical items from the HCR-20 were not able to predict institutional violence. They reasoned that the clients were, by definition, high risk, and therefore the historical scale was unable to discriminate between violent and nonviolent groups. Other sample and normative characteristics to consider include age range of your clients, mental health status, and point within the criminal justice process (e.g., pretrial, release, probation).

With regard to the purpose of assessment (research vs. clinical), research shows that clinicians tend to give lower ratings on risk appraisal instruments than do researchers (de Vogel & de Ruiter, 2004). This makes intuitive sense because the researcher will have little personal negative consequences for a liberal score, whereas a clinician faces the realities of contributing to the potential loss of liberties of the client and is likely to have his or her work scrutinized by supervisors, mental health professional peers, or cross-examined in a legal proceeding. The type of client (offender vs. civil vs. forensic) should also be considered. For example, the Brief Psychiatric Rating Scale has been found to be predictive of violence with a forensic sample (Gray et al., 2003), but not predictive of violence in the three-state MacArthur sample of civil psychiatric patients (Monahan et al., 2001).

Outcome Relevance

As noted above, it is unlikely that an instrument is going to directly address the outcome of interest. The closer the published validity studies of the risk appraisal instrument to the outcome of interest, the better. Significant advances have been made in this area. In fact, since Bonta's (2002) criticism that there were few instruments that directly measured criminal justice outcomes, the availability of criminal justice-related appraisal instruments has blossomed. As noted above, there has been great growth in the number of instruments applied to various offender samples; many of these provide sufficient psychometric properties and predictive validity to be used for risk appraisal. At this time, most risk appraisal instruments can predict general violence (Harris & Rice, 2003). However, outcome specialization has also occurred, with spousal abuse and sexual offending as good examples. Another consideration with outcome is the time frame that you are assessing. Ensuring that the risk appraisal instrument has shown validity for the time frame, whether brief or very long, is also important. Additionally, information regarding the context of where the potential violence is to occur is very important. Trying to use an instrument to predict violence in maximum security units will be greatly limited if you are using general community violence norms (Edens, 2006). Context can also have a role in community supervision. An offender with an intensive reporting structure will have different opportunities to reoffend than an offender reporting at less intensive intervals.

Actuarial Statistics

Communicating the results of a risk appraisal instrument's score is best done with probability and confidence intervals. Confidence intervals recognize the possibility of measurement error and assign a numeric estimate called the standard error of measurement (SEM). For example, if the observed score of an instrument was 20 and the SEM was 2, the confidence interval would be from 18 to 22, usually stated as "There is a 95% likelihood that the actual score lies between 18 and 22." A probability (e.g., offenders with similar scores reoffend at a rate of 20% over 2 years) communicates more information than does a descriptive category (e.g., low, moderate, or high). With probabilities a direct comparison can be made with rates of violence for other groups of scores (those higher or lower scores). Also the probability associated with a score can be compared to a different group, such as released offenders or the average incarcerated offender. These types of comparisons set the probability within a wider context, thereby improving the meaning that is communicated to the decision maker. This eliminates the vague characterization of low, moderate, and high risk.

Relevance to Risk Management/Intervention

One goal of conducting violence risk assessments is to provide guidance to reduce the future likelihood of violence (Einhorn, 1986). Given that crime and antisocial behavior are constantly in the public forum, most people have an opinion of what is needed to reduce criminal acts. For the clinician, just as for the layperson, the proffered opinion can be guided by factors other than those identified in the outcome literature on correctional treatment. For example, consider a client who lacks self-confidence in social situations and is easily influenced by others. Although the first instinct of many clinicians will be to recommend self-esteem enhancement treatment, the empirical literature suggests that a recommendation to increase self-esteem will not reduce criminal behavior and may possibly increase an individual's propensity to commit crime. A violence risk assessment with optimal accuracy offers little value-added information if the recommendations for managing risk are counterproductive. Thus, having an instrument that can assist in informing intervention from the evidence-based literature will make a significant contribution to the risk management process.

Given that no one variable in itself causes violence, it is prudent to use instruments that cover multiple domains (Bonta, 2002). These domains each need to be related to future violence and provide guidance for intervention. Most static/historically based instruments will not meet this criterion as the items measure some aspect of criminal history. There is also legal precedent to include multiple domains. In the *Sell v. United States* decision the court pointed out that important contextual variables were not assessed (Hunter, Ritchie, & Spaulding, 2005). The court found the assessment to be too narrow and indicated that the contextual variables of history and environment conditions are important in completing a risk assessment.

Relevance to Theory

Relevance to theory is not to be confused with relevance to risk management: measuring a theory or explanatory construct is different than identifying variables to provide guidance on risk management strategies. The use of a construct will assist in providing an explanation for the behavior. Specific areas of guidance may include substance abuse, but if risk estimates can be placed within a broader construct, such as attachment theory, then substance abuse can be used to explain how it disrupts attachments. However, construct validity, by itself, is not sufficient for selecting an instrument to use in violence risk assessments. With limited predictive validity the application of such an instrument in a risk assessment situation will require too great of an inference to the referral question or legal issues at hand (Otto & Heilbrun, 2002).

The utility of a risk assessment is greatly increased if the report can tell an explanative story (see Chapter 7). Telling an effective story involves communicating the understanding of why and how people chose to act out and commit crime. Also answering "Why certain events may happen in the future?" will be informative for the decision maker. Having an empirical basis for the story is helpful and allows the assessor to focus on improving public safety. To tell a good story it will be necessary to use multiple constructs (e.g., antisocial attitudes, antisocial associates, youth history, family situation, mental health issues, substance abuse). Some extrapolation needs to occur, so be careful. The more you extrapolate (i.e., go beyond the data) the more questionable your opinions, conclusions, and recommendations.

Some areas of caution are warranted. For example, extrapolation beyond the data is a caution that can be found with the PCL-R. Edens (2006) outlined three current views on psychopathy that have questionable support. First is the view "Once a psychopath, always a psychopath." A basic assumption is that psychopathy, by definition, is a dispositional construct. Some evidence for this is that those with high PCL-R scores tend to have significant childhood difficulties (Hare, 2003). However, Edens pointed out that there are no well-controlled longitudinal studies that have followed young psychopathic adults to determine if they remain highly psychopathic throughout the lifespan. Second is the view "Where the psychopath goes, violence is sure to follow." The PCL-R traditionally, both in the research literature and in the courts, has been associated with violence. Meta-analysis indicates a relationship between violence and the PCL-R (Walters, 2002), but this type of evidence does not mean that a particular psychopathic individual will become violent in the future. The third view, "Psychopaths are qualitatively different from other offenders," is based on the work of Harris and colleagues (Harris, Skilling, & Rice, 2001). They used a statistical technique developed by Paul Meehl to select a latent taxon, arguing that psychopaths are a discrete natural class. Edens, Marcus, et al. (2006) and others (Guay, Ruscio, Knight, & Hare, 2007) presented evidence that psychopaths may differ in degree rather than in kind. Given this evidence, caution is warranted when using terms such as "psychopathy" or "psychopathic traits" in a violence risk assessment.

Exposure to Criticism

Increased exposure can take several forms, including not being able to fully complete an instrument, potential difficulties under cross-examination, lack of transparency, or lack of training for using a specific instrument. If routine risk assessments are being conducted, then the information necessary to complete the risk appraisal instrument should be readily available. For example, if selection of a particular instrument will routinely result in missing information, you will unduly increase your exposure to criticism.

Instrument complexity also increases exposure to criticism. A more difficult instrument has the disadvantage of possibly contributing to more errors in either compiling the ratings or in the scoring of the scale. Simply stated, the more complex the instrument, the greater the potential for errors and instrument misuse. Research on scoring errors suggests this can be a substantial problem and can change outcomes for individual clients (McGrath,

2003). In addition to scoring errors, rater drift (i.e., ratings changing as a function of time; see Smith, 1986) can systematically contribute to different scores over time (i.e., decreased reliability including interrater reliability). Given that most risk instruments involve ratings, rater drift may gradually occur.

There are safeguards that clinicians can use to reduce the likelihood of instrument misuse. We recommend you consider these safeguards for your own protection as well as that of your client. First, scoring accuracy needs to be emphasized; the goal is high accuracy, even if the task has the appearance of being mundane or unimportant. Second, it is important to have the scoring manual with you *every time* you score the instrument. This procedural method allows you to state with greater certainty (as long as you actually consult the manual each and every time) that you take measures to ensure adherence to the scoring criteria. Under cross-examination it can always be questioned whether you followed the scoring criteria outlined for the instrument. Stating unequivocally that you consult the manual on each and every assessment will show that you have given this issue considerable care.

Third, obtain proper training. Nothing can replace appropriate training, so you must ensure that you have (or can attain) the necessary and proper training prior to using the appraisal instrument. Testing out a new instrument on clients to determine whether or not you should use the instrument is an unacceptable practice. If the instrument is complex, additional training may be warranted to ensure an adequate level of reliability.

Fourth, at set milestones, have another assessment clinician check your ratings and scoring. That is, you should develop a process of peer review of your instrument scoring, instrument interpretation, and report writing. This could occur at either a specific number of assessments (e.g., 15–20) or within a designated time frame (e.g., every 4–6 months). You might even choose to state this practice in your assessment procedure. Essentially this is a self-structured peer-review process which you may wish to have formally documented. Incorporating a formal periodic peer review may reduce your exposure when your assessment is called into question (which will eventually happen). At other times you may also want another clinician to look over your assessment, especially if the assessment involves a controversial or high-profile case. This need not be frequent, but is beneficial and ensures a higher level of confidence in these reports. Furthermore, this is not an uncommon practice in postdoctoral forensic fellowship training programs for both fellows and staff. If it is a valued learning exercise for doctoral-level trainees and trainers alike, it is likely a valuable learning experience for all clinicians engaged in this line of work. It should be noted that if you are informally involved in a peer-review relationship, you are strongly advised not to send your reports electronically to your colleague. The point of this exercise is to reduce your exposure, not to increase it, which any unencrypted electronic transfer will do.

Rating Scales versus Self-Report

Rating scales are purported to have the benefit of ensuring systematic coverage of an area and assessing symptoms (Myers & Winters, 2002). However, empirically, self-report and rating scales have roughly equal predictive validities. Among OMDs, Blackburn, Donnelly, Logan, and Renwick (2004) used a multimethod (self-report vs. interview), multitrait (personality disorders) methodology to examine which methods would account for a greater amount of the predictive relationship. Given the strong design, the results have a high level of generalizability. Both self-report and interview measures accounted for similar amounts of the relationship with personality disorders. In a similar comparison of self-report and interview-based ratings among non-mentally ill offenders we have found that the self-report of antisocial areas has the same validity as a rated instrument over a 9-year follow-up period (LSI-R; Kroner, Mills, & Morgan, 2007). This result is supported by Walters (2006), who conducted a meta-analysis comparing self-report and rated instruments. When using self-report instruments that contained crime-relevant content, both self-report and rated instruments predicted recidivism and institutional adjustment equally well.

Although there is substantial evidence that self-report instruments are as valid as rating instruments in routine assessments, we recommend the use of rating instruments. Before presenting our rationale for using rating instruments in routine risk assessments we acknowledge that self-report risk instruments serve an important purpose. Specifically, self-report instruments have strong utility as a screening measure. Screening can be helpful prior to an interview where an interview-based risk appraisal instrument will be scored. As with all psychometric self-report instruments, they serve to generate hypotheses that the clinician is expected to assess and test in the interview. In official proceedings, where social science ideals need to merge with legal deliberations, clinician ratings are the standard. A greater emphasis is placed on the role of the expert and the reliability and validity of the data source. In spite of evidence to the contrary, self-report is perceived as being of less value. Even though most self-report instruments have validity indices, this may not be sufficient when they are challenged during legal proceedings. Well-established instruments, such as the Millon Clinical Multiaxial Inventory III (MCMI-III; Millon, Davis, & Millon, 1997), may have problems with admissibility in court. In fact, some have argued that the MCMI-III does not meet the *Daubert* standard for Axis II disorders and therefore should not be used in assessments (Rogers, Salekin, & Sewell, 2000). You do not have to agree with this position to understand that validated self-report instruments may face difficulties in legal proceedings. Using rated instruments will likely reduce your exposure to this unwanted criticism.

PROFESSIONAL OVERRIDE?

As clinicians, it is tempting to believe that our integration of risk factors will improve accuracy. In other words, if we observe something that raises a concern with regard to risk, and the issue is not captured in our instrument of choice, we often invoke our professional prerogative that this information needs to be added to the actuarial estimate of risk. This falls within the realm of professional overrides. *Professional override* refers to the process of using clinical judgment to "override" actuarial data.

There are two types of professional overrides. One is an attempt to make the risk estimate more conservative and the other is to relax the risk estimate. Using a variable outside the risk instrument for a more conservative rating will decrease the mental health professional's predictive accuracy. In terms of decision-making errors, this is similar to a false positive, where a judgment is made that someone will be violent, when, in fact, he does not commit another violent act. Doing this with a predictive scale reduces the overall predictive accuracy.

Probably the most common situation that prompts a professional override is when the client indicates that he or she will do something in the future. With regard to these intentions, Hanson (1998) stated, "It would be foolish for an evaluator to dismiss an offender's stated intention to reoffend" (p. 61). Hart (1998) further questioned, "Does it matter at all what an offender's total score is on the VRAG ... if he also expresses genuine homicidal intent?" (p. 126). Borum and Reddy (2001) stated, "Base-rates of violent behavior for people who have engaged in foreboding, troublesome, or menacing behavior in the community and have not been subject to any intervention are typically not well documented" (p. 379). We would argue that stated intent, by itself, is not sufficient to change an actuarial risk estimate for general violence.

For example, consider a case where you are conducting a violence risk assessment on a client and you determine according to a risk appraisal instrument that the client's score suggests a 30% likelihood over a 3-year period. During the interview, the client informs you that when he is released he is going to "find and kill the person" that put him in prison. In such a circumstance, some highly regarded researchers have argued that this situation would call for a professional override, and the person should be considered a high risk to be violent. Here are some problems with this override approach. The risk appraisal instrument was designed to predict general violence (assault, robbery, etc.) against an unspecified target over a period of time. The threat the client expressed was a specific threat against a specific target with a relatively specific time frame. To "override" the actuarial estimate of risk is to mix outcomes and purpose. It would in effect equate the clinician's judgment of risk for violence toward a specific target to violence toward any target. We would argue that the client's risk for general violence against unspecified targets over 3 years remains moderate. However, the specific threat raises the issue of a duty to warn/protect of a *Tarasoff* nature. In this instance, as the clinician, you would have to consider the nature and credibility of the threat, the means available to carry out the threat, and so on (refer to our previous discussion regarding *Tarasoff*). Ultimately, two assessments would be undertaken and reported. One assessment would be the client's general risk for violence to society, which is one where actuarial estimates can be provided. The second assessment relates to the specific threat to a specific person. This assessment will always be clinical judgment as there are no actuarial estimates for a specified act against a specified target in a specified time frame. In a *Tarasoff* decision, the clinician is not making an assessment to predict an outcome (Thienhaus & Piasecki, 1998).

Changing a scale score, with appropriate evidence, is different than making a professional override. An example of changing a risk score based on appropriate evidence was demonstrated by Harris and Rice (2007a). Using the VRAG, they presented evidence that with the passage of time while successful on supervised release, the client could have his or her actuarial estimate of risk lowered. More specifically, the estimate of client risk could be lowered by one bin[1] after 10 years of successful supervision, and by another bin after 15 years of successful supervision. These reductions of risk did not occur with the passage of time during incarceration.

The second situation is encountered when the client does not appear to be as severe a risk as the results from the risk instrument suggest. In this situation the score is relaxed to the next lower category. This override is typically provided in situations where the client has undergone extensive treatment or intervention. More will be said on the influence of intervention in the next section.

There are two consequences of professional overrides. First, they reduce the predictive accuracy of assessment over time. There will always be those cases when our "additional information" (not captured by the risk appraisal instrument) appears to be the better predictor or at least alters the risk appraisal instrument, resulting in the perception of a more accurate prediction. One significant problem is the perception that the judgment was

---

[1]A cluster of scores associated with probability estimate. For example, scores on the VRAG from 0 to +6 are associated with a recidivism rate of 35% over 7 years. The next lower "bin" are scores from –7 to –1, which are associated with a recidivism rate of 17% over 7 years.

correct because very rarely do clinicians who complete violence risk assessments receive feedback on the success, or not, of the client. There are several other problems with using this type of experience to guide violence risk assessment. Hindsight bias, vivid factors, and our professional entitlement will contribute to the perception that case by case we will be able to improve prediction. There is no evidence indicating that professional overrides systematically improve prediction. Second, if we begin using professional overrides in routine assessments, the usage of them will likely increase over time. With the occurrence of this practice there will be a systematic undermining of the psychometric properties of the risk appraisal instrument. In our opinion, professional overrides have little utility in violence risk assessment.

ASSESSING CHANGE FROM INTERVENTION/TREATMENT

The issue of assessing treatment gain is one of the more difficult issues in risk assessment. Gendreau and colleagues call the assessment of change in risk a "key prediction issue" (Gendreau, Goggin, French, & Smith, 2006, p. 738). The courts have indicated that treatment gains need to be properly evaluated. In a 2004 case before the Superior Court of New Jersey Appellate Division (*In the Matter of the Civil Commitment of G.G.N.*, 2004), a psychiatric patient who had received 14 years of treatment was evaluated by two clinicians who did not take into account the potential treatment results. In the clinicians' assessment they were dismissive of treatment, but the appellate division ruled this practice unacceptable. Before addressing the specific issues in assessing treatment gain, one assumption needs to be met. That is, does treatment work? If this question cannot be answered, then the professional's opinion has the greater likelihood of being put into the "hearsay" category of evidence, which courts will have more difficulty finding admissible. The short answer to the above question is, yes, appropriate treatment with offenders does reduce recidivism.

The more complete answer is, on average, appropriate treatment, both in terms of content and mode of delivery, does work to reduce recidivism. Treating specific target areas that are directly related to crime-causing factors has a more consistent influence on reducing recidivism. After reviewing the current meta-analysis on correctional treatment, Lipsey and Cullen (2007) conclude that, with appropriate treatment, the preponderance of evidence suggests that recidivism can be reduced. The evidence suggests that even with a perceived recalcitrant group of psychopaths treatment can have a benefit. Using a sample of civil psychiatric patients, Skeem, Monahan, and Mulvey (2002) found that treatment for psychopaths can reduce violence. Specifically, they found that the more treatment involvement by those with psychopathic characteristics, the less likely they were to commit future violence. This treatment effect was strongest over the first 10 posttreatment weeks.

Using fear-based approaches in a specific deterrence framework does not work. "Specific deterrence" refers to the use of punishment to reduce subsequent criminal behavior. Examples of specific deterrence include shock probation and Scared Straight. Meta-analysis of Scared Straight programs (exposure to the frightening surroundings of incarceration) find that they actually increase recidivism (Aos, Phipps, Barnowski, & Lieb, 2001; Pestrosino, Turpin-Petrosino, & Buehler, 2003). In general, treatment programs that are predominantly emotionally based do not work. This includes focusing on an offender's self-esteem (Sherman et al., 1998).

Increased referral and monitoring in the community has little impact on reducing recidivism. If anything, because of the greater supervision, rates of reincarceration increase because there is greater opportunity to be caught. In their summary, Lipsey and Cullen (2007) concluded that increased supervision or other intermediate sanctions do not reduce recidivism. With regard to mode of delivery, less structure and nondirective approaches do not reduce recidivism with offenders (MacKenzie, 2000). However, the other extreme also has poor results. Programs that have excessive structure, discipline, and challenge as central components do not reduce recidivism. The meta-analyses on boot camps show no or minimal impact on recidivism (Aos et al., 2001; MacKenzie, 2001). Mixed results have been found when working with OMDs. Mental health court diversion programs, without addressing crime-causing variables in the treatment protocol, have shown minimal impact in reducing recidivism. However, with the inclusion of addressing crime-causing variables, mental health courts appear to effectively reduce recidivism (Moore & Hiday, 2006; McNiel & Binder, 2007).

When listing nonempirical theories of crime, Gendreau and colleagues (Gendreau et al., 2006; Latessa, Cullen, & Gendreau, 2002) colorfully present treatment endeavors that are not tied to criminal outcomes as "correctional quackery." Examples of correctional quackery include acupuncture, haircuts and diets, heart mapping, healing lodges, horticulture therapy, been there–done that therapy, drama therapy, pet therapy, sage smudging, and yoga. Although these are extreme examples, the point taken is that if clinicians are not tying interventions to criminal risk factors, they are providing inappropriate services (i.e., quackery).

In contrast to the above strategies, programs using positive interactions and supporting constructive change aimed at crime-related factors are often successful in reducing recidivism (Lipsey & Cullen, 2007). Those interventions with high structure, that have a cognitive-behavioral approach, and that are delivered in the community (compared with institutional settings) have the most success (Andrews et al., 1990; Gendreau et al., 2006). This conclusion is based on hundreds of studies, across many settings, with various methodologies. With regard to content, Andrews and colleagues have found that addressing antisocial attitudes, antisocial personality, antisocial associates, family relations, substance abuse, and impulsiveness are most important (Andrews et al., 1990). Similarly, focusing on antisocial attitudes, family processes, and antisocial associates is effective in reducing recidivism among female offenders (Dowden & Andrews, 1999).

In addition to style and content, a third area of effective offender treatment is program integrity. In a meta-analysis, Andrews and Dowden (2005) examined which integrity variables contributed to reduced recidivism. The most important variables were trained staff, with clinician supervision, and when the researcher was involved. Other integrity variables such as include manual use, monitor change, and provide adequate dosage (number of sessions or exposure to treatment modules) distinguished the appropriate treatment from the nonappropriate treatment.

Thus, the first step when assessing for the possibility of treatment gain is to determine if the client was in a program that had the potential to reduce recidivism. Three areas outlined below need to be addressed. These areas include a focus on the principles of change rather than on a specific technique or trademarked therapy. Rosen and Davison (2003) point out the benefits of using principles to describe treatment interventions. A focus on principles allows one to draw upon the psychological literature for evaluating the effectiveness of new programs. Not relying on psychological principles of intervention would require that every new twist to a treatment approach would have to be fully evaluated, which is not practically possible. For example, Rosen and Davison noted that even established programs that are principles-based, such as Marsha Linehan's dialectical behavior therapy (DBT), should drop components that are not necessary for positive outcomes. The shift from specific treatments to principles also allows for the decision rules to become simpler. By using the three principle for evaluating interventions outlined below, the question is not which programs are better (i.e., more effective) than other programs, but whether these principles of effective intervention are present? The more of these three principles you meet, the more likely your program will prove beneficial for reducing recidivism.

1. *Supportive therapeutic efforts.* Was the program focused on positive interactions and supportive constructive change? Any indication of "putting offenders in their place," provoking offenders to anger that was similar to their offense, or breaking offenders down emotionally results in a negative treatment response. Such strategies are generally less effective and negate this principle regardless of what other positive strategies were utilized.

2. *Content tied to criminal risk factors.* The primary treatment content

must include risk factors empirically tied to criminal behavior, such as anti-social attitudes, antisocial personality, antisocial associates, family relations, educational and occupational functioning, leisure and recreational pursuits, substance abuse, and impulsiveness.

3. *Program offers a high level of treatment integrity.* Programs that ensure treatment integrity are more effective. Therefore, determine the following: Was adequate staff training available, was clinician supervision provided, were treatment process and outcome measures incorporated into the treatment program, was there a structured treatment manual available to enhance treatment integrity, and did the program ensure adequate treatment dosage?

Second, you will need to determine if there is evidence of change within your client. This evidence will come in three forms. Behavioral evidence of change in the context that is being predicted will be the strongest evidence that change has occurred, allowing for a stronger causal statement of treatment change. Although behavioral assessment is optimal, there are not many assessment situations that will afford a clinician this type of data.

The next strongest evidence will be behavioral evidence, in a similar, but different context. For example, if a treatment program occurred within a prison, and 6 months passed prior to conducting a release assessment, then the 6-month period could be used as evidence for behavioral change resulting from the treatment targets. Some caution is necessary because the structure of prison places greater constraints upon a person than does the community.

A more common scenario of assessing treatment change is conducting the assessment at the end of a treatment program. The assessment is then used for a decision-making function (e.g., reduction in security level, release to the community, reduced supervision requirements). With this type of assessment, the timing of the assessment may preclude any type of behavioral evidence of treatment change. Having pre- and posttesting may be helpful if the test directly measures treatment constructs and the above three questions are satisfied. This is a weaker form of evidence because measuring pre–post change has been strongly debated by methodologists (Zumbo, 1999).

The above are issues that need to be considered to determine whether your client has *potentially* benefited from treatment. However, even with the above criteria fully satisfied, it is unlikely that you will be able to categorically determine that your client has benefited from treatment. Specifically, we know of no way to determine empirically that a specific individual's risk has been reduced because of treatment benefits. There are two primary reasons for this. The first is that much of the current treatment outcome research emphasizes pre–post group differences on content measures, that is to say, that outcome studies that examine recidivism are not as routine as they ought to be. Second, the psychometric issue of accurate measurement is still in its infancy. In the correctional treatment literature the pre–postdifferences in content measures rarely relate to an outcome measure of recidivism. When treatment differences are related to an outcome measure, the effect sizes are small and usually do not replicate. Gendreau et al. (2006) indicated that the lack of measures that allow for the measurement of change is a pitfall in criminal justice research. Also, the correctional treatment literature has put a large amount of effort into the aggregate benefits of treatment such as those reported by Andrews and Bonta (2006) who aggregated 374 effect sizes and Lipsey and Cullen (2007) who reviewed solely meta-analytic treatment studies. Little effort has been put into determining how to identify which person has benefited from treatment. Therefore, at the present time, it is possible to identify treatment programs that have the qualities necessary to effect change and potentially reduce recidivism, but there is no way apart from group membership (the client took the program) to extrapolate if the program reduced the client's likelihood to reoffend.

THE PERCEPTION AND COMMUNICATION OF RISK INFORMATION

Perceiving Risk

The communication of risk information is arguably the least studied aspect of violence risk assessment. Evaluating risk communication within government agencies was among the top three areas identified as a priority for research by experts both within academia and government agencies (Chess, Salomone, & Hance, 1995). Despite the call for research into violence risk communication within the contexts of forensic risk assessment nearly 10 years ago (Heilbrun, Dvoskin, et al., 1999), there has been very little research reported within the literature. Taking lessons from weather forecasting, Monahan and Steadman argued in 1996 that risk assessment in the field of forensic mental health was considerably lacking. At the end of their review they concluded that the research focus to that point was in producing accurate risk estimates and not in the effective communication of those estimates. What modest forensic research that has been conducted to date has examined how professionals communicate risk as well as how professionals understand or perceive risk. This latter focus on the perception of risk information should logically precede the study of how to communicate the risk information.

    In other disciplines, much research has gone into understanding how people perceive societal risks. Research over the past 30 years has shown that experts tend to view risk from societal hazards differently from lay-persons. Typically, experts view risk in terms of fatalities based upon technical estimates, whereas laypersons consider other societal issues such as the potential for catastrophe (Slovic, Fischoff, & Lichtenstein, 1984). Other areas of science have recognized this diversity of risk perception and have called on scientists to recognize these differences and promote dialogue between scientists, decision makers, and stakeholders (Renn, 2004).

One important publication that helped to define how the public responds to hazards was written by Paul Slovic. In his 1987 work published in *Science*, Slovic studied 81 diverse societal hazards that ranged from the innocuous, such as use of elevators, to the more sinister, such as nerve gas accidents and radioactive waste. These hazards were rated on 18 risk characteristics such as a person's fear of them and how controllable and observable the hazard was. These ratings were subjected to an analysis that showed that the public generally viewed hazards along two continuums. The first was their "Dread" of the hazard and the second was how "Unknown" was the risk of the hazard. Other similar analysis specifically included such hazards as terrorism and crime (Slovic, Fischhoff, & Lichtenstein, 1982). These hazards were found to be high on the "Dread" continuum and were perceived to have relatively known consequences. Our own work studied this two-dimensional perception of risk specifically with different types of crime (Mills et al., 2010). We confirmed that different criminal offenses varied along both the Dread and the Unknown continuums and as with Slovic and colleagues' (1982) findings they tended to be high on Dread and the consequences were perceived to be generally known. Further, the types of crime we investigated were perceived in terms of Dread in an order similar to the same crimes' judged dangerousness in other research (Howe, 1994).

Laypeople view as relatively more dangerous those individuals who commit more severe crimes (whether property or interpersonal), those who commit interpersonal crimes over property crimes, and those who are repeat offenders over those who are first-time offenders (Sanderson, Zanna, & Darley, 2000). Laypeople also show an intrinsic knowledge that repeat offenders are more likely to reoffend than are first-time offenders.

Research on the Communication of Risk Information

For nonforensic groups and issues, preferences as to how to communicate risk information are unclear. Some participants prefer numerical and some verbal reports, though there appears to be a willingness to change depending upon the nature of the information being conveyed (Wallsten, Budescu, Zwick, & Kemp. 1993). Those who prefer numerical communication cite its accuracy as the primary reason for this preference, while those who prefer verbal communication cite ease as the primary reason. Monahan and

Steadman (1996) noted in their review that the public seems to prefer probabilistic information over qualitative statements. They argued in favor of numerical statements but also indicated that there was importance in the inclusion of other descriptive or qualifying information.

A survey asked clinicians trained in conducting forensic risk evaluations how they communicated their risk findings (Heilbrun, Philipson, Berman, & Warren, 1999). Only 1 in 55 reported that they used numerical figures. When asked why probability statements were not used, nearly half reported that the scientific literature did not justify using specific numbers. When asked what their stated preferences were, there was no majority opinion. The most reported method was to identify how specific risk factors may raise or lower risk; this method was followed closely by the use of descriptive categories such as low, moderate, and high. In a second and similar study, 90% of clinician participants reportedly did not use numerical probabilities to report risk. In this latter study participant ratings indicated a preference for providing clinical impressions based on history and current behavior and then describing how specific risk factors raise and lower risk.

Previous research has focused on the comparison of prediction (risk estimation alone) versus risk management models of risk assessment (Heilbrun, 1997). As we have already stated (see Chapter 1), we do not view these two as disparate approaches but rather as essential to a comprehensive assessment of risk which has also been described as a broader definition of risk assessment (Heilbrun, 2003). When prediction and management approaches are dichotomized and the preferences of professionals are sought, some trends become apparent. Overall, the most valued form of risk communication was the identification of risk factors and strategies to reduce the risk (Heilbrun, O'Neill, Strohman, Bowman, & Philipson, 2000). With closer scrutiny predictive styles are preferred when only static information is available and a risk management style is preferred when dynamic risk factor information is available (Heilbrun et al., 2004). This would suggest that the clinicians who conducted the ratings matched the type of information provided with the risk communication style that best suited the type of information. Other research by Zoe Hilton and colleagues (2005) showed that the inclusion of risk-relevant information in a vignette in conjunction with a summary statement that included a numerical estimate of risk tended to result in inflated estimates of risk. This suggests that the respondents may be somehow adding their own perception of the risk factors to that of the actuarial estimate which had already included those risk factors in the estimate.

There has been some research into the method of risk communication. For example, there is more than one way to communicate the likelihood to reoffend. One study compared the use of probabilities (i.e., 10%) with frequencies (i.e., 1 out of 10) among clinicians and generally found that those individuals who were asked to rate cases using frequencies rated overall risk as lower (21.1 out of 100) than those who were asked to rate the same cases using percentages (30.2%) (Slovic, Monahan, & MacGregor, 2000). In a follow-up study described in the same report, these researchers found that educational material regarding what was meant by harm and probability and what constituted good risk assessment did not alter the phenomenon. In yet a third study with clinician participants, Slovic and colleagues (2000) found that those clinicians who were presented with percentages tended to rate as lower risk the same scenario when compared with those clinicians who were presented with frequencies. The same tendency for frequencies to be perceived as higher risk was replicated by Monahan and colleagues (Monahan et al., 2002), but work by Hilton et al. (2006) did not find a significant difference in risk estimates between frequency and probability statements. In addition more vivid portrayals of the crime also lead to more conservative decision making but only for those clinician participants who worked within forensic facilities (Monahan et al., 2002).

In addition to finding differences in how risk is perceived between risks represented as probabilities versus frequencies, research has found that the perception of risk can be altered by changing the range of options (Slovic & Monahan, 1995; Slovic et al., 2000). For example, by limiting the choices by having the highest category of risk equaling "> 40%," both clinicians and laypeople estimated risk to be lower than when they were provided options ranging from 0 to 100%. In addition it was determined that individuals perceive dangerousness in a stepwise fashion. That is to say, that once the perceived risk of a case exceeds a threshold, the rater perceives the individual to be "dangerous." However, the threshold for dangerousness varies quite considerably among raters.

Our own work in this area of risk perception has shown that clinicians, like laypeople, tend to overestimate the rates of violent and sexual crime, even when base rate information has been provided (Mills & Kroner, 2006b). Clinicians who were explicitly provided base rate information did not differ from clinicians who were not provided base rate information on their estimate of violence and sexual recidivism rates. There appeared to be a tendency for clinicians to rate moderate risk at around the 50% mark regardless of the base rate. For example, even when told that the base rate was 30% for violence, clinicians still rated 50% as "moderate" for violence. Later in a follow-up study we examined what happened when we explained base rate to naive (student) participants. We discovered that with an explanation, student participants rated estimates of violent and sexual crime lower than those who had no base rate (Mills et al., 2010). In addition to findings that demonstrate that professionals show substantial disagreement in their understanding of descriptive risk categories, these nonnumerical or descriptive risk categories have also been shown to be subject to the effect of context (Hilton, Carter, Harris, & Sharpe, 2008). Together, this work shows the susceptibility of descriptive categories to incorrect interpretation in the communication of risk. To simply say low, moderate, or high risk leaves the consumer of the assessment in a quandary as to what that information means and the research suggests that he or she will overestimate the rate of recidivism. If one combines the use of descriptive categories with the identification of specific risk factors, which Hilton et al. (2005) suggests inflates risk estimates, then risk is likely to be perceived as still higher. These reasons contribute to our position that wherever possible risk assessments should be anchored by a statistical risk estimate.

Risk and Decision Making

Interestingly, structured and unstructured approaches to the evaluation of risk were experimentally compared using simulated offender information (Samra-Grewal, Pfeifer, & Ogloff, 2000). There was no meaningful difference in their conclusions between methods for both professionals and nonprofessionals engaged in the task. A part of the structured process was the use of a table of risk categories. While the participants arrived at the correct risk classification, it did not seem to have any bearing on their ultimate decision whether to grant parole; hence, their decisions were similar to those participants who did not have the benefit of the structured approach. Also, specific factors differed in terms of the variables that contributed to a positive versus a negative decision. For those granted a release, the key factors were the offender's participation in and benefit from treatment programs and the offender's proposed release plans. For those who decided to deny release, the offenders' understanding of and attitude toward their criminal behavior was the central factor.

Review boards have a poor track record of making release decisions based on actuarial risk information. In Canada, offenders who receive a determinate sentence (not life) are generally released on community supervision after serving two-thirds of their sentence. In cases in which the risk is determined to be unmanageable, an offender can be detained beyond the two-thirds date. Patricia Nugent (2000) compared offenders who were detained by the National Parole Board in Canada with offenders who were not detained and released on their two-thirds statutorily determined release date. Her study showed that detained offenders were significantly lower in terms of actuarial risk as determined by the SIR-R1 (see Chapter 3) and not significantly different in terms of risk as measured by the VRAG and the LSI-R. The resulting Hit Rate (% of true predictions) for the parole board was 35% for general recidivism and 18% for violent recidivism, whereas utilizing the SIR would have resulted in a Hit Rate of 69% for general recidivism and 63% for violent recidivism.

One of the most convincing studies that indicates that the bane of violence risk assessment are often decision-making boards was conducted by Zoe Hilton and Janet Simmons (2001). These authors examined 187 decisions made by review boards in cases of maximum security male forensic hospital patients. It is important to note that the setting was the same one where the VRAG was developed and had been used for a number of years in the decision-making process. A number of patient variables were examined in relation to the decisions. These variables included IQ, psychopathy as scored from the PCL-R, the patients' status (i.e., insanity acquittee or not criminally responsible), and patient attractiveness. Other variables included length of stay, prior admissions, index offense, criminal history, VRAG score, institutional management problems, active psychotic symptoms, life skills deficits, senior clinician's testimony, and multidisciplinary team recommendation. These researchers examined what characteristics were correlated with the review board's decision. Strong associations were found between the senior clinician's testimony and the multidisciplinary teams' recommendation and the review board's decision. There was no association between the VRAG (actuarial risk measure) and the review board's decision. There was also no association between the VRAG score and either the clinician testimony or team recommendations.

Given the importance of the senior clinician's testimony and the team recommendation, a follow-up analysis examined which variables predicted these outcomes. The variables that best predicted both of these outcomes included institutional management problems, medication compliance, patient attractiveness, and criminal history. Most notably, risk for violent recidivism as measured by the VRAG did not contribute to either clinician testimony or team recommendation. What appears to be happening in these instances is the following. Risk assessment has focused on the structured assessment of risk variables to ensure reliable and valid measurement. These variables are then combined in a structured or algorithmic manner to produce a score that is either quantified in the case of an actuarial application (%) or qualified in the case of SPJ. Note that to this point the risk information is governed by guidelines. This risk information is then handed over to the decision makers who then treat it as one piece of information in their overall clinical judgment. This risk information is then only a part of the decision process and other variables such as good behavior and attractiveness enter (we would argue unwittingly) into the decision makers final edict. Hence, all of the work and energy put into the fidelity of the assessment process is lost when the ultimate decision is made. The decision makers lapse back into first-generation "clinical decision making."

The Challenge of Communicating Risk

The challenge that faces every clinician involved in risk assessment is how to effectively communicate the risk information that is available. We agree with Kirk Heilbrun and colleagues who observed that "the translation of nomothetic empirical data into idiographic conclusions regarding a single individual has proved to be one of the more difficult challenges in violence risk assessment as well as for decision making on other issues" (Heilbrun et al., 2000, p. 140). In light of the research, what is the best strategy for communicating risk?

Given the evidence, using an actuarial estimate wherever possible is the essential first step. At first blush this may appear as a statement that rules out the use of SPJ instruments but it is not the case. We are wholly convinced that simply reporting descriptive categories of low, moderate, or high is not sufficient, though an all-too-common practice. We are equally convinced that a lone statistic is better, but still not sufficient to convey risk information. We see three central components to effective risk communication: first, establishing an actuarial risk estimate within the context of group norms; second, identifying central risk factors with particular emphasis on dynamic risk factors; and third, identifying intervention and risk management strategies that can potentially moderate that risk.

Actuarial Risk Estimates

The actuarial risk estimate is simply that—an estimate. Oddly, clinicians have been reluctant to use actuarial risk because they do not feel it can be that precise (see Heilbrun et al., 1999). Actuarial estimates are probability statements that should be characterized as such. It is intrinsic to a probability estimate that an individual shares the characteristics of a *group* that has a specified likelihood (e.g., 40%) to reoffend within a specified time frame (e.g., 3 years). This also means that within three years 60% of that group will not reoffend. This does not mean that a specific person in the group *has* a 40% likelihood to reoffend but rather that he or she shares characteristics with individuals who as a group, it is estimated that 40% will reoffend. Also, the probability associated with the group is an estimate. This means that it may change from sample to sample and outcome to outcome. It is an estimate. That is why it is also important to place the estimate within the context of the group as a whole. That is to say that identifying an individual as belonging to a group of whom 40% are likely to reoffend within 3 years should be placed within the context of the base rate (call it an average within your report) of the sample on which the estimate is based. This provides the decision maker with the anchor of the average rate of recidivism against which to measure the individual.

Different instruments communicate risk in different ways. For example, the RRASOR and the Static-99 associate a probability with a single score, whereas the LSI-R and the VRAG associate a probability with a group of scores (which we will refer to as a "bin"). For example, scores on the LSI-R from 24 to 33 are associated with a 48% likelihood to reoffend. Some individuals have problems specifying a single probability as they know that there are such things as *SEMs*. This is true of all instruments but likely affects instruments that require clinical assessment such as the VRAG and LSI-R more than instruments that are purely based on official static/historical information such as the Static-99. One conundrum associated with this problem is that of an individual's score falling on the border between two risk categories. Most clinicians know from their training with other measures that a specific score has error attached to it. For example, if an individual's score fell on the upper limit of a particular risk category, it is reasonable to rate the person's risk as likely between $X\%$ (the category they fell in) and $Y\%$ (the next category up). This approach reflects the scientific knowledge that there is error in measurement and that risk is being estimated.

It is also important to specify the time frame to which the risk estimate refers. Some instruments, as you have seen, provide multiple time frames and others only a single time frame. Risk estimates change with time, with the greatest rates of recidivism occurring within the first 12 to 18 months. Also, it is important to define what you are predicting and be as specific as possible. This is particularly important when assessing crimes of low occurrence such as murder. If you are assessing an individual who has committed murder and are asked to provide an assessment for the propensity for violence, the subtext that is not spoken is really what is the individual's likelihood to commit murder again? Of the risk appraisal instruments that we are familiar with, none have murder among the outcome criteria (to the best of our knowledge). Most violent occurrences are assaults and robberies of varying degrees of severity. Even if there were a single murder among the many outcomes in the sample of development, it would indeed be a stretch to suggest that the outcome you are predicting includes murder. Therefore in these types of cases it is important to be clear to what the estimate you are providing is really referring.

Identifying Central Risk Factors

Depending upon the instrument that you use, identifying risk factors can be more or less transparent. For example, if you employed the LSI-R, most of the central risk factors are identified within the instrument. There may be other risk factors specific to the case but they are not included in the instrument. Instruments such as the Static-99 are based more upon historical risk factors and therefore your knowledge of the more dynamic risk factors becomes all that more important as you will need to identify not only historical issues but also the dynamic or changeable risk factors that are evident in the case. These other risk factors are found in the literature (see Chapter 2) but they are also found in other risk instruments. We are not suggesting the use of multiple instruments, as you will note from our earlier discussion, but those instruments may contain important dynamic variables that you can identify as a point of intervention or management. This is also a good point to interject the reminder that identifying additional risk factors does not automatically mean an increase in risk per se. As we discussed previously, due to multicollinearity (see Chapter 3), many of the dynamic risk factors are highly related to the static factors already considered in the actuarial estimate.

Identifying Intervention and Risk Management Strategies

Once the central risk factors have been identified it is appropriate to identify what types of intervention or management strategy would assist in managing the case. This would include possible treatment within an institution or within the community. Your knowledge of the local criminal justice and mental health settings will play an important role at this point in the assessment process. The Risk–Need–Responsivity principle (Andrews & Bonta, 2003) will be a good model to follow at this point in your assessment. Simply put, the higher the level of risk, the more resources are necessary to manage the case. Also, "need" here refers to those dynamic or potentially changeable risk factors that could be addressed through intervention and are associated with (or explain) the level of risk. "Responsivity" refers to individual issues that may influence how intervention and risk are managed, such as intellectual functioning or serious mental health issues.

Intervention and management strategies can be very broad. These strategies may include such things as the *amount* and *duration* of supervision. Generally more supervision is required for higher risk cases. They can include treatment or program groups to deal with specific issues such as substance abuse, anger and emotions management, criminal associates, and criminal thinking. They may also include more individual intervention such as employment counseling, housing, and mental health services. The time frames for interventions should also be considered. That is, determine what interventions should be accomplished before release and what interventions could be accomplished in the community. Of course all of these possibilities must be considered in light of the individual. Persons with mental illness may not be capable of sitting through a traditional program or intervention. Likewise an individual with limited cognitive abilities may also not be able to function within traditional group interventions. Both of these specific individual differences may also require a modified approach to supervision, which should be detailed as necessary.

As we mentioned, knowledge of what resources are available in terms of intervention and management is essential. Listing comprehensive interventions for which there is no hope of attainment due to existing resources will only serve to suggest that the individual's risk is not manageable. On this we cannot offer concrete advice as jurisdictions vary considerably in terms of resources available to intervene. It will be important for you to find a balance where you do your best to provide a solid intervention and risk management strategy to adequately manage the risk and public safety while at the same time not burden the individual and the system with impossible requirements.

In this chapter we covered a number of issues that serve to make the violence risk assessment process a challenge. We hope it has become evident that there are multiple issues, each with its own challenges and requirements for special knowledge in order to be adequately addressed. Choosing a risk appraisal instrument has increased in complexity if for no other reason than the clinician needs to understand the options available and make a rational empirically based decision he or she can defend when choosing a risk appraisal instrument. Professional overrides to actuarial findings are tempting and there are many examples where this is undertaken. We reported on what we believe are the problems with this practice as the clinician needs to understand the potential issues he or she may encounter in court where he or she has to explain his or her actions or possibly rebut the actions of others who took a different approach and arrived at a different conclusion. Assessing the potential for change intersects the professional override issue in that both call for an alteration to actuarial conclusions. Change is theoretical until proven and proving change is difficult with the current state of construct and behavior measurement. In addition to these challenges is the effective communication of the risk assessment findings. Research in this area of violence risk assessment is wanting, yet it is at the very point in the process where all of the assessment efforts are applied. Despite these very real challenges violence risk assessment can be successfully undertaken and provide useful information to decision makers. The following chapter focuses on the integrated–actuarial approach to violence risk assessment.

CHAPTER 5

■   ■   ■

AN INTEGRATED–ACTUARIAL APPROACH TO THE ASSESSMENT AND MANAGEMENT OF RISK FOR VIOLENCE

We have defined the term *integrated–actuarial risk assessment* to refer to the integration of (1) actuarial risk estimates within the context of group norms, with (2) potentially dynamic risk factors, (3) intervention/ treatment recommendations, and (4) risk management strategies. Integrating these elements has been recommended for some time now. Steadman et al. (1994) observed that "risk assessment without risk management leads only to dichotomous 'in–out' judgments for institutionalization without much relevance for clinical practice" (p. 298), and "risk management without risk assessment ... is not directly responsive to the concerns of mental health law" (p. 299). Steadman et al. concluded that including risk management strategies added potentially dynamic factors related to the individual's functioning and likelihood for violence over time to the assessment process. Similarly, Heilbrun et al. (1998) argued for the integration of risk assessment, intervention, and decision making as part of the overall risk enterprise. Elsewhere, Doyle and Dolan (2002) suggested integrating information from actuarial, clinical, and structured clinical sources to create a formulation for the management of risk. Taken together, the integrated–actuarial approach is viewed as a best practice by many with expertise in risk assessment. This chapter outlines how you can take this approach using different risk appraisal instruments.

ANCHORING THE ASSESSMENT
WITH ACTUARIAL ESTIMATES

As we noted in Chapter 1, actuarial risk estimates have been shown to consistently outperform clinical judgment. So we recommend that you start by anchoring your assessment with an actuarially based instrument and communicating, where possible, a risk estimate using a probabilistic statement (e.g., "40% of individuals with a similar number of risk factors commit violent acts over a 3-year period"). As we discussed in Chapter 4, be careful how you communicate risk information in the report. Specifically, when you present actuarial estimates, provide as well some parameters for understanding them, lest readers of your report draw faulty conclusions. First, and most importantly, your report should note that the individual him- or herself does not have a 40% chance to reoffend, but rather that he or she shares risk characteristics with a group of offenders of whom 40% will reoffend within a given period of time. Clinicians, juries, parole officers, and judges may misconstrue statistics presented in forensic reports—assuming a statement about a "40% risk" means there is a 40% chance the person you assessed will reoffend. In your report, be sure you avoid creating this misperception. Second, your report should specify the type of violence it is predicting. For example, is the violence general criminal violence, spousal violence, or sexual violence? In most studies, "violence" includes a broad range of behaviors, from pushing and shoving to instrumental robbery to serious and life-threatening attacks. As we have already noted, if a client is serving a sentence for homicide, the question on the mind of the decision maker is generally, "Will this person kill again?" Actuarial risk instruments cannot predict the likelihood of this specific type of violence (e.g., murder) over the long term, and your report needs to make that clear. Third, the outcome being predicted is based upon *detected* recidivism. It is generally accepted that detected (officially recorded or adjudicated) violence is generally below the number of actual violent acts perpetrated (see Monahan et al., 2001). Fourth, your report should specify a time frame for the predicted violence. Research indicates that longer term follow-ups (e.g., 6 years) tend to produce greater rates of detected violence (Harris & Rice, 2007a). Fifth, whenever possible, the average recidivism rate for the comparison group should be reported. This average provides the decision maker with an anchor by which to judge the relative risk of the individual. As we have already noted, there is a tendency when descriptive approaches are used for the person reading the report to overestimate the likelihood to reoffend (Mills, Green, Kroner, & Morgan, 2010).

INTEGRATING DYNAMIC FACTORS FOR INTERVENTION/ TREATMENT AND RISK MANAGEMENT PURPOSES

From our earlier review of the advances in risk assessment, you will recall that a number of researchers are attempting to measure dynamic change in violence risk factors. If they are successful in measuring such changes in risk factors, these measurements will enable us to make more precise estimates of actuarial risks—what we have referred to as a "dynamic–actuarial risk assessment." Although researchers are on the cusp of making dynamic–actuarial risk assessment the preferred approach, prospective replications are years away. Retrospective studies are not nearly as helpful when looking at changes in dynamic risk factors because of the measurement bias in these types of studies. Hence advances in this form of risk assessment will likely take much longer because of the need for prospective studies. There have been a number of recent prospective studies that have examined changes in dynamic risk factors and found them to be related to risk for recidivism.

Quinsey, Book, and Skilling (2004) examined a number of dynamic variables in a sample of mentally retarded psychiatric patients who had been released to the community. Their findings showed more success at discriminating between violent and nonviolent patients (between patients) than discriminating when a patient would be violent (within patients). In other words, clinician ratings are better at predicting who might engage in antisocial behavior over predicting when a violent behavior may occur. Those dynamic variables that discriminated between violent and nonviolent patients include inappropriate and antisocial behaviors, dynamic antisociality (e.g., takes no responsibility for behavior, sees him-/herself as victim, blames others), poor compliance (with supervision), and medication noncompliance/ dysphoria. Trend analyses showed a deterioration in performance from the 6 months prior to a violent incident, to the month prior, and then to the month of the violent incident to be significant for the dynamic variables of psychotic behaviors and inappropriate and antisocial behaviors.

Quinsey et al. (2006) followed a large group of forensic psychiatric patients for an average of 33 months. Each month, they assessed a number of potentially dynamic variables in the patients. The researchers identified those patients who failed in some way (antisocial or criminal behavior) and compared the ratings taken in the month in which an incident took place (the index month), with the month prior to the index month (prior month), and the average ratings of the 6 months before the prior month (previous months). In this way they could identify the within-person variables that were related to the incident. Changes in a number of variables between the index month and the immediately prior month were related to outcome: psychotic behaviors, dynamic antisociality, psychiatric symptoms, poor compliance, medication noncompliance/dysphoria, denies all problems, and therapeutic alliance. For a more conservative estimate of changes related to an incident these researchers considered differences between the average of the previous six months with ratings of the month prior to the index month because these two ratings could not be contaminated with hindsight bias as the raters did not know at the time the individual was about to fail. These comparisons yielded fewer significant relationships; the only factors that were significantly related to outcome were dynamic antisociality, poor compliance, and therapeutic alliance. Variables where change was related to a violent incident specifically included inappropriate behaviors and therapeutic alliance. This research demonstrates that while the content represented by certain risk factors may be related to recidivism, measuring change in those risk factors and relating them to outcome is much more difficult.

Other studies have examined changes in risk factors for recidivism more broadly defined. In a study of risk factors among aboriginal (North American Native) offenders in Canada, offenders were assessed both upon admission and at termination of their probation (Bonta et al., 1997). Changes in these risk factors were correlated with recidivism, and for nonaboriginal and Métis (aboriginal) offenders the relationship was significant. More recently, a multiwave study of dynamic risk variables that measured dynamic risk factors once prior to release, and then 1 month and 3 months following release, demonstrated that in general, dynamic risk factors tended to improve among the successful offenders over time (Brown, St. Amand, & Zamble, 2009).

Identifying dynamic risk factors is not the same as indicating which specific individuals will be violent in the presence of that risk factor. For example, Jennifer Skeem and colleagues examined the *contextualized* (violence in the presence of a specific context) prediction of violence among hospital patients (Skeem, Mulvey, & Lidz, 2000). Clinicians were asked to predict which patients would be more likely to be violent if they had been drinking. Follow-up with these patients found that clinicians could identify those who would be violent, though the effect size was quite modest. Clinicians tended to predict in general that the patients who drank heavily were more likely to be violent when drinking, and that patients who drank more were more likely to be violent. However, they were unsuccessful in identifying which patients would be more violent when they had been drinking.

From our review in Chapter 2 you will recall that both static and potentially dynamic risk factors were identified for a number of violent outcomes. Other sources of potentially dynamic risk factors that are measured in a structured manner may come from risk appraisal instruments that incorporate dynamic variables specifically such as the Stable-2007 and the Acute-2007 for sexual violence, the LSI-R and the HCR-20 for general violence, and the SARA for spousal violence.

Once you have identified dynamic risk factors, the next step is to incorporate these risk factors into the risk assessment process. When you are using a dynamic–actuarial approach, clearly delineate the incorporation of the dynamic risk factors and how they relate to the actuarial estimate of risk. In most other circumstances, when an integrated–actuarial approach is being used, remember that the dynamic risk factors do not alter actuarial risk estimates. Rather treatment/intervention and appropriate risk management strategies for these dynamic risk factors become the focus.

In cases where certain dynamic risk factors are central to the assessment of risk and those risk factors are not represented in the actuarial risk appraisal instrument, some authors recommend that you adjust the estimate through a descriptive caveat. For example, the authors of the Static-99 Coding Rules (Harris et al., 2003) have suggested the following possible wording in such cases.

> "Based on a review of other risk factors in this case I believe that this STATIC-99 score (Over/Under/Fairly) represents Mr. X's risk at this time. The other risk factors considered that lead me to this conclusion were the following: Stable Variables: Intimacy Deficits, Social Influences, Attitudes Supportive of Sexual Assault, Sexual Self-Regulation, and General Self-Regulation; Acute Variables: Substance Abuse, Negative Mood, Anger/Hostility, Opportunities for Victim Access—Taken from the SONAR (Hanson & Harris, 2001)." (p. 71)

There are at least three problems with this approach. First, violence risk factors are multicollinear. In other words, risk factors are intercorrelated: individuals who score high on one risk factor tend to score high on other risk factors (see Chapter 3). Those with a history of violent behavior tend to abuse substances and to have interpersonal relationship problems. Consider as a hypothetical example a risk appraisal instrument that measured "history of violence" and "substance abuse" but not "interpersonal relationship problems" or "personality disorder." We know that all of these risk factors are related to future violence and that all these risk factors are intercorrelated. We also know that adding risk factors to a predictive equation yields progressively smaller increments of predictive information. If you were assessing a client who had interpersonal relationship problems, and used a scale that did not measure this risk factor, it would be tempting to adjust the actuarial finding (i.e., most likely, you would report a higher risk than the scale indicated). The inherent problem with this approach is that you do not know *if* or *by how much* the risk factor of "relationship problems" is improving on the actuarial estimate or predictive accuracy of the instrument you used.

The second problem with allowing such adjustments in our opinion is that later evaluations may make similar adjustments, but base them on a different risk factor—one that will have a different salience to you and to the consumer of your risk assessment. This introduces unsystematic information into the actuarial estimate that becomes "noise" in the risk assessment process. The third problem is that not all relevant but unincluded risk factors are dynamic; some are static. The same argument for adjusting estimates based on absent dynamic risk factors holds for adjustments based on absent static risk factors.

If dynamic risk factors change over time—and we argue that you should not adjust actuarial estimates based on risk factors not included in the risk appraisal instrument—then how do you include potentially dynamic risk factors within the risk assessment process?

Dynamic or changeable risk factors have more potential to explain behavior than do static risk factors. Consider as an example the risk factor of substance abuse. Some people have a history of being violent only when intoxicated, and in such cases substance abuse may explain violence through reducing inhibition to violent acting out. For other people, antisocial associates or gang affiliation may explain much of their violent behavior. As will become apparent when we discuss the risk assessment report, explaining an assessed person's behavior may be as important—if not more so—as providing a simple probability of the client's likelihood to reoffend. Both substance abuse and criminal associates are modifiable risk factors and are therefore considered to be potentially dynamic. Both, therefore, could be the subject of treatment or intervention such as substance abuse treatment groups or through programs to address antisocial attitudes and associates. Both could also be the target of restriction during a community release through special conditions to abstain from alcohol use or refrain from associating with known criminal offenders. Both could also be used by individuals supervising these clients as indicators of risk that require intervention when observed. In the next section we provide an example of how to integrate both actuarial estimates and dynamic risk factors.

THE TWO-TIERED VIOLENCE RISK ESTIMATES SCALE: AN INTEGRATED–ACTUARIAL APPROACH

As an example of how to integrate actuarial estimates with risk management strategies, we will use an instrument called the Two-Tiered Violence

---

[1]The TTV items and scoring are reproduced here with the permission of the authors.

Risk Estimates[1] Scale (TTV; Mills & Kroner, 2005). We developed the TTV to help integrate the clinical functions of assessing risk and communicating it (report writing). As such the TTV comprises the Actuarial Risk Estimate (ARE), which provides a statistical estimate of risk, and the Risk Management Indicators (RMI), which provides a structured assessment of risk factors associated with violent recidivism that have the potential to change over time. The TTV integrates the actuarial prediction of violence likelihood with the assessment of dynamic factors through structured clinical judgment. This assessment approach is consistent with what we described in Chapter 1 as an *integrated–actuarial approach.* Integrating these two methods allows you to establish an underlying risk for violence, recommend points of possible intervention to manage the risk, and monitor potential changes in dynamic risk factors. Out of these dynamic or changeable violence risk variables, intervention and risk management strategies can be developed and varied as changes occur with the client over time. This risk management approach to risk assessment and communication is consistent with the method preferred by forensic clinicians in which risk factors are identified and interventions stated (Heilbrun et al., 2000).

The TTV ARE comprises 10 historical items that will not change during the client's sentence or hospitalization (see Table 5.1). Some items may increase once the client has been released to the community and has the opportunity to incur further charges. However, the TTV RMI are designed

TABLE 5.1. Items of the TTV

ARE: 10 items	RMI: 13 items
1. Childhood antisocial behavior	1. Employment
2. Adolescent antisocial behavior	2. Financial
3. Age of first adult conviction	3. Substance abuse
4. Prior incarcerations	4. Mental health issues
5. Prior convictions for assaultive behavior	5. Family instability
6. Community supervision failure	6. Associates
7. History of alcohol abuse	7. Attitudes
8. Failure to complete high school	8. Leisure
9. Criminal associations	9. Resistance to intervention
10. Interpersonal difficulties	10. Mood
	11. Social support
	12. Environment
	13. Stressors

so they can be measured on more than one occasion, providing ongoing information on changes to violence risk variables.

Development and Psychometric Properties of the TTV

The TTV was developed based upon a retrospective study of risk factors associated with violence in a sample of predominantly violent offenders serving 2 years or more in a Canadian penitentiary. Range (0–13), mean (M = 8.3), and standard deviation (SD = 3.3) of the ARE's scores were calculated based on a sample of 247 male offenders. The ARE's standard error of measurement is based on the intraclass correlation coefficients of similar instruments used on a portion of this sample (see Kroner & Mills, 2001) and found to approximate .90. The SEM, therefore, of the TTV ARE is approximated at 1.04. The SEM will become important when the probability of violence is estimated for the client.

Based on our retrospective construction sample, the TTV ARE is strongly correlated with other existing measures of both violent and general recidivism (Table 5.2). AUC was employed as an index of predictive accuracy and the ARE was found to be consistent with other measures (Table 5.3).

The base rates for reoffending in this sample were 48.8% for general recidivism and 29% for violent recidivism. The number of days to an act of general recidivism ranged from 6 to 1,566 (M = 331.4, SD = 348), and the number of days to an act of violent recidivism ranged from 6 to 1,566 (M = 423.8, SD = 396). The days of opportunity for nonrecidivists ranged from 25 to 2,209 (M = 1108.4, SD = 506.6). This represents an average follow-up period approximating 3 years.

TABLE 5.2. Comparative Correlations between the ARE, Other Risk Appraisal Instruments, and Recidivism

	ARE	Violent recidivism	General recidivism
ARE	—	.32***	.39***
PCL-R	.68	.18**	.27***
Factor 1	.31	.13	.13
Factor 2	.69	.12	.24**
LSI-R	.79	.26***	.39***
VRAG	.67	.26***	.38***
SIR	.84	.30***	.39***

Note. PCL-R, Psychopathy Checklist—Revised; LSI-R, Level of Service Inventory—Revised; VRAG, Violence Risk Appraisal Guide; SIR, Statistical Information on Recidivism.

**p < .01; ***p < .001.

TABLE 5.3. Comparative AUCs between the ARE and Other Risk Appraisal Instruments and Recidivism

	Violent recidivism	General recidivism
ARE	.698	.718
PCL-R	.616	.653
Factor 1	.592	.585
Factor 2	.571	.632
LSI-R	.682	.734
VRAG	.675	.721
SIR	.684	.719

Note. PCL-R, Psychopathy Checklist—Revised; LSI-R, Level of Service Inventory—Revised; VRAG, Violence Risk Appraisal Guide; SIR, Statistical Information on Recidivism.

Subsequent to the original construction study a second concurrent validity study was undertaken to examine the relationship of the TTV with existing risk assessment instruments (Cheston, Mills, & Kroner, 2007). The participants were 61 male offenders. The mean age of the participants was 42.6 years (*SD* = 13.4). The racial composition of participants was predominantly Caucasian (82%) and they were incarcerated for violent offenses (86%). In addition to the TTV, the HCR-20, the LSI-R, and the PCL-R were all scored concurrently by the same rater.

The ARE mean is quite consistent with the ARE mean of the original construction sample on which the TTV was developed (current study ARE = 8.3, original study ARE = 8.3). The correlations between the TTV scales and the other risk appraisal instruments were quite strong.

Correlations between the instruments are consistent with the underlying purpose of the TTV (see Table 5.4). Both TTV measures are not related to Facet 1 (Interpersonal) or Facet 2 (Affective) of the PCL-R but are both strongly related to Facet 3 (Lifestyle) and Facet 4 (Antisocial). Facets 1 and 2 comprise the personality component of the PCL-R (Factor 1) and Facets 3 and 4 comprise the antisocial lifestyle and history or Factor 2 of the PCL-R. It is the latter Factor 2 of the PCL-R that is most consistently related to antisocial behavior and violence. Both TTV measures are strongly and equally related to the LSI-R. This is not unexpected, as the LSI-R combines both historical and dynamic factors within one lengthy measure. Some divergent validity appears evident in the relationship of the TTV measures with the HCR-20. The TTV ARE is more strongly related to the H-10 (Historical items) than to the TTV RMI, whereas the R-5

TABLE 5.4. Correlations of the TTV with Concurrent Measures of Risk

	ARE	RMI
ARE	—	.61***
RMI	.61***	—
PCL-R	.47**	.46**
Facet 1 Interpersonal	−.04	.05
Facet 2 Affective	.07	.14
Facet 3 Lifestyle	.57***	.62***
Facet 4 Antisocial	.69***	.40*
LSI-R	.77***	.77***
HCR-20	.82***	.72***
H-10	.85***	.59***
C-5	.59***	.64***
R-5	.33*	.62***

*$p < .05$; **$p < .01$; ***$p < .001$.

(Risk Management items) of the HCR-20 are more strongly related to the TTV RMI than to the TTV ARE. Taken together there is evidence for the validity of the TTV ARE and RMI. The next section outlines how to score these instruments.

Actuarial Risk Estimates Scoring Protocol

The TTV actuarial risk variables are scored on the basis of the offender's history prior to arrest (if a pretrial assessment) or incarceration. These variables in one form or another are common to other risk schemes because they have been shown to be effective predictors across a variety of populations. Scoring of these variables should be done on the basis of both interview and official file or court information. Users are encouraged to consult the scoring directions for each use and not assume that they have remembered the instructions correctly.

A1. Childhood Antisocial Behavior

This variable is scored on the basis of the individual's behavior up to the age of 12 years. Consider all sources of information related to the person's behavior at home, at school, and in the community. Look for the presence of fighting; running away from home; criminal activities; early sexual activity; bullying; problems with authority figures such as teachers, parents, and police; substance abuse (alcohol and drugs); difficulties in school such as truancy and class disruption—particularly resulting in suspensions or expulsions. An official diagnosis of conduct disorder would suffice to score this item. This item is scored dichotomously as present or not present. This item should be scored as present if the antisocial behavior is persistent across time. A single or a couple of relatively minor incidents that are considered average developmental experiences or that are situational in nature would not warrant an endorsement of this item.

Childhood antisocial behavior not present   0
Childhood antisocial behavior present   1

A2. Adolescent Antisocial Behavior

This item references the individual's behavior between the ages of 13 and 17 years. This item refers to any behavior that resulted or could have resulted in an arrest. If the individual admits to criminal behavior for which he was not arrested (e.g., breaking and entering for which he was not caught) then the criteria for this item would be considered met. A single or a couple of relatively minor incidents that are considered average developmental experiences or that are situational in nature would not warrant an endorsement of this item.

No adolescent antisocial behavior   0
Adolescent antisocial behavior   1

A3. Age of First Adult Conviction (Both Felony and Misdemeanor)

To score this item, determine the age at which the offender was first convicted as an adult (18 years of age and above)

Age 31 or more   0
Age 20–30   1
Age 18 or 19   2

A4. Prior Incarcerations

To score this item, determine the number of times that the offender has received a period of incarceration as a disposition of his sentence. The score should include juvenile or young offender incarcerations if known. Detention upon arrest is not included.

No prior incarcerations   0
1–3 prior incarcerations   1
4+ prior incarcerations   2

A5. Prior Convictions for Assaultive Behavior

Scoring this item requires the identification of all convictions (including juvenile) for crimes that involve the assault of another person. Included would be crimes of homicide, aggravated assault, sexual assault, assault causing bodily harm, and simple assault. Robbery in which a physical assault took place (e.g., aggravated robbery) would be included.

No prior assaultive convictions   0
1–3 prior assaultive convictions   1
4+ prior assaultive convictions   2

A6. Community Supervision Failure

This item refers to a failure on a form of conditional community release. These would include bail, probation, parole, statutory release, or any form of release where residing in the community is conditional on good behavior and meeting certain conditions. Failure on community supervision would include incurring new offenses or breaching conditions of release regardless if the failure resulted in charges.

No community supervision failure   0
Prior community supervision failure   1

A7. History of Alcohol Abuse

This item refers to the individual's prior abuse of alcohol. Evidence for prior abuse should include a pattern of excessive drinking that may or may not have resulted in criminal charges. The presence of charges that resulted from alcohol abuse would meet the criteria. Abuse is indicated if the individual's drinking resulted in problems in one or more life areas such as relationships, school, employment, and so on. A prior diagnosis of alcohol abuse or dependence would meet the criteria for this item.

No history of alcohol abuse   0
History of alcohol abuse   1

A8. Failure to Complete High School

To score this item, identify if the individual completed high school during the usual adolescent period of life. Jurisdictions may vary in terms of the number of years or what the grade level is called; therefore, completion of high school requirements within the individual's social jurisdiction is the criteria. Brief breaks in high school education due to specific circumstances such as illness would not count against the individual. Leaving high school and returning as an adult or upgrading to complete (e.g., General Equivalency Diploma) do not meet the criteria of having completed high school.

Completed high school	0
Did not complete high school	1

A9. Criminal Associations

To score this item determine if the individual regularly associated with anyone who has a criminal record or who has committed acts that would constitute criminal behavior. These would include close friends, associates, and family members.

No criminal associations	0
Criminal associations	1

A10. Interpersonal Difficulties

This item refers to chronic instability in interpersonal relationships. This item refers primarily to intimate and/or cohabiting (nonintimate) relationships. The focus of this item is on the nature of the relationships, specifically has there been regular or ongoing conflict in the relationship(s)? If the individual is single and does not report problems in intimate relationships, then this would be scored a zero.

No relationship difficulties	0
Relationship difficulties	1

Calculating the TTV ARE

To calculate the TTV ARE, score the 10 items using the scoring form found in Figure 5.1. For each item place the correct numerical value in the column on the far right of the page. Add the resulting 10 numbers together for a total. Risk estimates and their confidence intervals (plus and minus 1 around the score) should be transposed to the TTV scoring form.

Actuarial Variable	Scoring		Score
A1. Childhood antisocial behavior	Childhood antisocial behavior not present	0	
	Childhood antisocial behavior present	1	
A2. Adolescent antisocial behavior	No adolescent antisocial behavior	0	
	Adolescent antisocial behavior	1	
A3. Age of first adult conviction	Age 31 or more	0	
	Age 20–30	1	
	Age 18 or 19	2	
A4. Prior incarcerations	No prior incarcerations	0	
	1–3 prior incarcerations	1	
	4+ prior incarcerations	2	
A5. Prior convictions for assaultive behavior	No prior assaultive convictions	0	
	1–3 prior assaultive convictions	1	
	4+ prior assaultive convictions	2	
A6. Community supervision failure	No community supervision failure	0	
	Prior community supervision failure	1	
A7. History of alcohol abuse	No history of alcohol abuse	0	
	History of alcohol abuse	1	
A8. Failure to complete high school	Completed high school	0	
	Did not complete high school	1	
A9. Criminal associations	No criminal associations	0	
	Criminal associations	1	
A10. Interpersonal difficulties	No relationship difficulties	0	
	Relationship difficulties	1	
		ARE Total Score	

TTV Actuarial Estimate	Bounded score	1 year	2 years	3 years
Lower-bound ARE Total Score –1				
Upper-bound ARE Total Score +1				

FIGURE 5.1. TTV ARE scoring form.

Interpreting the TTV ARE

Incorporating time into prediction can be statistically accomplished with the Cox regression survival analysis. This statistic produces a probabilities curve as a function of time. An additional benefit of using Cox regression analysis is that it can produce an estimate of risk over time for each score of an appraisal instrument. This approach contrasts with traditional methods of risk estimation which limits the classification of instrument scores into three to five predictive categories. For example, the LSI-R has five categories of risk varying according to score (scores of 0–13 equal low risk [11.7%], scores of 14–23 equal low/moderate risk [31.1%], etc.). Using predictive categories to attribute risk has a number of difficulties not the least of which is a substantial change in risk between the two numbers on either side of a category cutoff point (e.g., a score of 13 or 14 on the LSI-R). Associating probabilities with each score on a risk appraisal instrument is a more idiographic approach to risk assessment.

Determining Level of Risk

Once you have calculated the TTV ARE total, locate the number in the far left column of Table 5.5. Recall that the *SEM* for the TTV is ±1. Therefore, we have a 95% confidence level that the individual's score lies from −1 to +1 around the score. By subtracting 1 from the score you get the lower bound probability and by adding 1 to the score you get the upper bound probability.

For example, if a client had a score of 6, then 5 would be the lower bound probability and 7 would be the upper bound probability. From Table 5.5 you will see that a score of 5 is associated with a recidivism rate of 5.5% for 1 year and 9% for 3 years, and a score of 7 is associated with a score of 9.5% in 1 year and 15.5% in 3 years. Since the Cox regression provides the likelihood of reoffending over time the risk of violent reoffending would be said to be *"between 5.5% to 9% within the first year following release*

TABLE 5.5. TTV ARE Violent Recidivism Actuarial Table (% Likelihood to Reoffend Violently)

TTV score	6 months	1 year	2 years	3 years
0	1	1.5	2.5	2.5
1	1	2	3	3.5
2	1.5	2.5	4	4.5
3	2	3.5	5	5.5
4	2.5	4.5	6.5	7.5
5	3.5	5.5	8.5	9.5
6	4.5	7	10.5	12
7	5.5	9	13.5	15.5
8	7.5	12	17.5	19.5
9	9.5	15	22	24
10	12	19	28	31
11	15	24	34	38
12	19	30	42	46
13	24	37	50	55

and increase to between 9.5% and 15.5% by the end of 3 years following release."

TTV RMI Scoring Protocol

The TTV's RMI were developed to guide the rater's identification of potential problem areas and facilitate recommendations of intervention strategies. These variables are scored on a 3-point scale: Not present (0), Present and requires monitoring/assistance (1), Present and requires intervention (2) (see Figure 5.2). The purpose of scoring these items in this manner was to focus the attention on the need for monitoring/assistance or intervention if present. The distinction between the latter two definitions depends upon the degree to which the risk factor has been addressed and is being adequately managed. Specifically, if a risk factor is present but the client has undergone an intervention to treat the risk factor (group work, programs, therapy) and the behavioral indicators are in abeyance or nominal, then we would conclude that the risk factor is present and requires monitoring/assistance. When the behavioral indicators are in abeyance monitoring would be indi-

Risk Management Indicator	Not Present (0)	Present and requires monitoring/ assistance (1)	Present and requires intervention (2)
M1. Employment			
M2. Financial			
M3. Substance abuse			
M4. Mental health			
M5. Family instability			
M6. Associates			
M7. Attitudes			
M8. Leisure			
M9. Resistance to intervention			
M10. Mood			
M11. Social support			
M12. Environment			
M13. Stressors			

FIGURE 5.2. TTV RMI scoring form.

cated, whereas behavioral indicators that are nominal would suggest presence of the risk factor where the assistance of the client (cooperative intervention and encouragement; working alliance with the client) is deemed most appropriate. In situations where the risk factor is present but interventions have been refused or not undertaken or where the behavioral indicators of the risk factor tend to be extreme, then the appropriate response is "intervention required." This may mean intervention while in custody or it may mean a tightening of supervision and more authoritative control if the client is in the community. Becoming involved in intervention may also be a contingency for possible release.

M1. Employment

Employment as a Risk Management variable focuses on the individual's commitment to seeking and securing employment commensurate with their ability.

Not present (0): If the individual is employed in a full-time capacity then this item would be scored as 0. If the individual is supported by a disability pension and/or is legitimately unable to work or can only work reduced hours, then this item would be scored 0.

Present and requires monitoring/assistance (1): If the individual is employed on a part-time basis and is capable of full-time work then this item is scored as 1 (present). An individual who is unemployed and seeking employment would be scored as having this Risk Management variable present.

Present and requires intervention (2): Severity of this variable may be considered high if the individual is unemployed and unwilling to seek employment. This would apply to those individuals who avoid work and earn money through criminal means.

M2. Financial

Finances as a Risk Management variable focuses on the individual's ability to manage and provide for basic needs on a day-to-day basis. A basic need refers to shelter, food, clothing, and daily incidentals.

Not present (0): Those individuals who are working or on a pension and are managing to meet their financial needs would be scored as 0.

Present and requires monitoring/assistance (1): If a person is having difficulty meeting his or her financial obligations through legitimate sources of income then this Risk Management variable is considered present. Indications of this would be use of food banks, unpaid bills, being behind in the rent, and the like.

Present and requires intervention (2): Individuals with little or no source of income, who are relying heavily on others for survival, would be considered to have severe financial difficulties. Homeless individuals also fit into this category.

M3. Substance Abuse

Not present (0): Individuals who score 0 on this variable are those with no history of substance abuse.

Present and requires monitoring/assistance (1): Those individuals who have a history of substance abuse but are at the present time not using substances still require support in terms of relapse prevention and support systems within the community and therefore this item is considered present.

Present and requires intervention (2): For those individuals who have a history of substance abuse and who are currently using substances, this item would be considered present and severe, requiring immediate intervention.

M4. Mental Health

The focus of this item is on the more chronic or recurring mental health issues. This item does not refer to individuals who have had only brief contacts with a mental health professional in the past for situational factors (e.g., a life crisis). Mental health issues for the purpose of this item refer to periods where the individual required intervention for psychotic disorders or mental illnesses related to mood such as depression, anxiety, or bipolar disorder. Mental retardation is also considered under this item.

Not present (0): No history of nor current symptoms of mental illness.

Present and requires monitoring/assistance (1): This item is considered present if the person has a history of mental illness defined above or if the person is currently in the care of a psychologist, psychiatrist, or physician and receiving intervention (medication or therapy) for mental health issues.

Present and requires intervention (2): This item would be considered acute if the mental health issues are currently impeding the individual's day-to-day functioning. This would include clinical symptoms (e.g., depression, anxiety) that would limit the activity of the individual.

M5. Family Instability

This item refers primarily to intimate relationships between cohabiting adults. However, it would also apply to individuals who reside in a halfway house and their partners in the community or to adults who are involved in an intimate relationship but living apart. In some cases the adult may not have an intimate relationship but is living with parents in a conflictual relationship. The focus of this item is on the nature of the relationship, specifically is there regular or ongoing conflict in the relationship? Conflict in these relationships contributes considerably to negative emotion and instability in living arrangements.

Not present (0): The individual is involved in an intimate or family relationship that is generally supportive and free from ongoing conflict.

Present and requires monitoring/assistance (1): The individual is involved in a family relationship that is not supportive or positive. He or she reports some conflict resulting in arguments or periods of separation.

Present and requires intervention (2): The individual is reporting constant conflict and daily arguing. Any evidence of physical assault or threats from either party in the relationship would constitute an acute problem.

M6. Associates

This item refers to the antisocial or criminal people that the client associates with in his or her free time. It does include family members. It is not the number of criminal individuals that matters most, it is if there are any criminal individuals within the client's association.

Not present (0): None of the client's associations include individuals who have a criminal record or who are currently involved in criminal behavior.

Present and requires monitoring/assistance (1): This item is scored as present if there is anyone with whom the client associates in his or her free time who has a criminal record or is involved in criminal behavior. Members of the client's family who have a criminal record or who are involved in criminal activity are included.

Present and requires intervention (2): The client has more than one relationship with a criminal or antisocial other and/or spends considerable time in the criminal milieu.

M7. Attitudes

The focus of this item is upon the client's overarching attitudes toward society's laws and conventions, particularly as they relate to violent behavior. This is often reflected in how he or she views his or her own criminal behavior. For example, does the client accept what he or she did was wrong with little or no excuses.

Not present (0): The client holds prosocial views and attitudes and considers antisocial and criminal behavior to be wrong.

Present and requires monitoring/assistance (1): The client holds attitudes that endorse antisocial behavior. He or she may excuse or legitimize the use of violence if provoked.

Present and requires intervention (2): The client is openly antagonistic to the law and social convention. The client identifies criminal activity as a legitimate though illegal method of earning a living.

M8. Leisure

This item refers to how the client spends his or her free time. Look for examples of productive leisure activities versus unstructured idle time.

Not present (0): The client has structured activities such as hobbies or sports that he or she regularly participate in or he or she spends his or her spare time actively parenting or in the company of prosocial family members.

Present and requires monitoring/assistance (1): The client spends his or her leisure time in an unstructured and unproductive manner. Look for examples of just hanging out with friends, watching excessive TV, or "listening to music." This is particularly important when the client is not employed and has much free time.

Present and requires intervention (2): The client has excessive free time (unemployed or on a pension) and cannot or does not account for any of the time in productive pursuits.

M9. Resistance to Intervention

Compliance with Intervention refers to the client's willingness to take direction and accept intervention that is directed toward managing risk or treating risk factors or mental health issues.

Not present (0): The client has accepted direction and participated in treatment as recommended. He or she has complied with medication regimes to improve mental health functioning. He or she has complied with or expressed a willingness to comply with conditions of release.

Present and require monitoring/assistance (1): The client has not participated in treatment as recommended. This is due to the client's decision and not circumstances that have kept him or her from participating. The client has not taken medication as directed or has not complied with conditions of release. Look for missed appointments in the community.

Present and requires intervention (2): Similar to the above description but the client is also openly antagonistic toward the authorities giving direction and continues despite being disciplined for noncompliance.

M10. Mood

Negative mood states have been shown to relate to recidivism (Quinsey et al., 2006; Zamble & Quinsey, 1997). This item refers to a negative change in the overall affective functioning of the client. The mood states of anger, sadness, and anxiety are of particular note. What this item focuses on is the increase in negative mood states. Changes in mood should be relative to the overall functioning of the client.

Not present (0): The client presents with generally stable mood. Occasional dysphoria or anger should not be significant or long-lasting.

Present and requires monitoring/assistance (1): The client has shown deterioration in his or her mood. Anger, sadness, or anxiety is more prominent than previously observed. The presence of these negative affect states need not reach clinical significance but represent deterioration from normal functioning.

Present and requires intervention (2): This item would be considered acute if it is present as described above and the emotions are strong and of immediate concern.

M11. Social Support

Social support refers to both professional and nonprofessional support systems available to the client in the community. Consider the client's overall need level when scoring this item. For example, a client with mental health issues will require both personal and professional support in the community, whereas a client without mental health issues who has strong family support would not necessarily require professional help.

Not present (0): This item would not be considered present if the client has social support systems, family and friends, who can assist him or her in the community

Present and requires monitoring/assistance (1): This item would be considered present if either personal supports are absent or professional supports are absent when necessary.

Present and requires intervention (2): This item would be considered acute if the client has no social supports at all or if the client's needs are extreme and the social supports are few and inadequate.

M12. Environment

This item refers to the environment that the client is returning to or living in. Specifically, is the client returning to an environment that is considered a high-crime neighborhood or to the same geographic area that was closely tied to his or her criminal activity?

Not present (0): The client is returning to or living in a neighborhood that does not have a high rate of crime or is not related to his or her criminal offending.

Present and requires monitoring/assistance (1): The client is returning to or living in a neighborhood that is known to have a high crime rate or is the same neighborhood that he or she came from that had an influence on his or her offending.

Present and requires intervention (2): This item would be considered acute if the client is returning to or living in a neighborhood that is known to have a high crime rate or is the same neighborhood that he or she came from that had an influence on his or her offending and the environment limits professional services, employment opportunities, or supervision.

M13. Stressors

This item refers to the day-to-day stressors experienced by the client. It should include significant changes, hassles, and difficulties. It should also be scored in relationship to the client's ability to cope with stressors. For example, a client with good coping ability and extensive social supports may be better able to cope with stressors than another client with fewer coping strategies and supports.

Not present (0): Stressors are well within the client's ability to cope and do not exceed what is expected day-to-day.

Present and requires monitoring/assistance (1): Stressors are present and are taxing the client's ability to cope. The client may express frustration, an absence of task-oriented solutions, and/or hopelessness at his or her situation.

Present and requires intervention (2): The item is present as described above and the client appears to be overwhelmed by life difficulties.

Once you have assessed the client on the RMI the results will serve to guide your recommendations regarding possible treatment to address relevant risk factors. For example, if you determine that the client has a history of alcohol abuse (see Figure 5.2, Item M3) and has been abstaining from alcohol use, then you may find the alcohol abuse to be in abeyance (present and requires monitoring/assistance). This is difficult to assess if the client is incarcerated. If the alcohol abuse is historic and has not been present for some time and the client has completed a substance abuse program, then monitoring would be in order. If the alcohol treatment has not occurred, then assistance (i.e., treatment) is recommended. On the other hand, clients who continue to use/abuse alcohol would warrant a rating of intervention; this means that intervention needs to occur now to manage/reduce risk. The same process will help you identify risk factors, which if they occur during release would require immediate intervention. For example, a client may have completed an alcohol treatment program and be maintaining sobriety at present; however, you may deem it necessary for immediate intervention should he or she return to alcohol abuse. This intervention may be administrative, such as suspending a release, or it may be therapeutic, such as a caution and referral to treatment. In this instance, substance abuse would be rated "present and requires monitoring/assistance," with the added observation that a return to substance use would warrant a change to "requires intervention."

OTHER EXAMPLES
OF INTEGRATED–ACTUARIAL RISK ASSESSMENT

As we have already stated, the use of the TTV-ARE at the present time should be limited to correctional clients. Efforts are under way in a prospective study to verify its validity with other populations. Even among correctional offenders, other actuarial instruments could be substituted for the ARE. For example, the SIR and the LSI-R (see Chapter 3) could be used to derive an actuarial estimate of risk in conjunction with the TTV's RMI.

The TTV's RMI are, however, consistent with risk factors for offenders with mental disorders and may be of use as a risk management tool in conjunction with an actuarial instrument such as the VRAG with these offenders. In such cases, the VRAG would provide the clinician with the actuarial estimate of risk and the TTV RMI would assist in the intervention and risk management portion of the assessment. The point is to simply ensure that in the assessment of risk you have an actuarial estimate for violence and a structured method to assist you in identifying potentially dynamic risk factors that can guide your recommendations for intervention and risk management strategies.

Applying an integrated–actuarial approach to sexual violence could be accomplished by using the Static-99 to establish an actuarial estimate of risk in combination with the potentially dynamic risk factors associated with

---

TABLE 5.6. Potentially Dynamic Risk Indicators for Sexual Violence

- Sexual preoccupation
- Lonely/single
- Behaviorally impulsive
- Emotional dysregulation/hostility/anger
- Emotional identification with children
- Antisocial orientation/peers
- Intimacy deficits/relationship instability
- Access to victims
- Uncooperative/noncompliant

sexual violence identified previously (see Table 5.6). Still better yet would be to receive training in the use of the Static-99, the Stable-2007, and the Acute-2007 and be able to integrate these static and dynamic variables in a truly dynamic–actuarial fashion.

Assessing spousal violence using the integrated actuarial approach would indicate the use of the ODARA in conjunction with the potentially dynamic risk factors identified in Chapter 2 (see Table 5.7).

INTERVENTIONS TO REDUCE RISK

This approach to assessing risk factors underscores our own bias in terms of how to consider the possible effect of interventions designed to reduce risk. A central difficulty in determining the efficacy of any treatment or intervention is selection bias. Most program evaluations do not meet a randomized design standard. As a result, more compliant and lower risk participants may complete a program, whereas high-risk and contrary clients may be more likely to fail (reoffend during the program) or simply opt not to attend or complete the program. For one example, spousal abusers who completed a 14-session treatment program reoffended at a lower rate than those who failed to complete the program (Hendricks et al., 2006). However, this study's definition of failure to complete the program included both reoffending and refusing to enter the program. This kind of bias is more a problem for evaluators who are trying to determine the efficacy of a program and obtain an accurate index of the actual effect of treatment. For the clinician, generally speaking, completion of an effective program is an indicator of a *potential* for risk reduction. We underscore potential, as thus far reductions of risk are imputed to the individual because of membership in a group (treatment completion) and not to specific changes in the individual that can be tied to a reduction in likelihood to reoffend. Even membership in a group of compliant and treated individuals does not suggest necessarily that the individual client's risk has been reduced.

TABLE 5.7. Potentially Dynamic Risk Indicators for Spousal Violence

- Substance abuse
- Behaviorally impulsive
- Emotional dysregulation/hostility/anger/jealousy
- Violation of noncontact orders/uncooperative/noncompliant
- Relationship instability
- Stalking spouse
- Perpetrator being unemployed

The integrated–actuarial approach to violence risk assessment can accommodate any validated actuarial risk appraisal instrument. Empirical information taken together with potentially dynamic factors serves to identify risk for violence within a normative context, and also the points for intervention, treatment, and risk management in the community. With future research dynamic–actuarial risk assessment will become more prominent, but only if it includes specialized training, given the importance of construct measurement at the item (individual-risk-factor) level. Having reviewed the risk factors, the more prominent risk appraisal instruments, related issues in risk assessment, and now a process for integrating risk factors, the next step is to outline a risk assessment *process,* which is essential to ensure a comprehensive and consistent approach to the evaluation of the potential for violence risk.

CHAPTER 6

■ ■ ■

THE RISK ASSESSMENT PROCESS

TRANSPARENCY

The approach you take when conducting a violence risk assessment has to be transparent. By that we mean a consumer of your report should be able to determine exactly what steps you took, what information you deemed central, what instruments you used, and how you arrived at your conclusions. This approach makes for a more defensible assessment, particularly if much time has passed since you conducted the assessment. Depending on your area of practice you may write assessments that are routinely considered in a judicial or a quasi-judicial setting, and you may not be called to defend those assessments often if at all. However, we would encourage you to make every assessment you write one that you are confident you can defend under cross-examination. We know colleagues who have been called to defend assessments 10 years after they wrote them. An approach that utilizes the principle of transparency will make it much easier for you to recall, explain, and defend the report.

Part of transparency should include a documented process for conducting risk assessments. You may wish to employ a checklist to ensure that elements of the process are not overlooked (we have included a sample checklist in Figure 6.1). A checklist is likely to be more important if there are more than one or two people involved in the assessment process. We advocate a standardization of the process and an a priori rationale for the selection of risk appraisal instruments in various risk assessment situations. Through a standardized approach you are using the same metric to measure different cases. Use will increase your competence with those measures and will eventually save you time. Further, once you have chosen a rational and

Terms of Assessment	
For whom: Who is the client?	
Who is the person to be assessed?	
For which violent outcome(s) is this requested?	
For what decision/proceeding is this assessment requested?	
Consent	
Competency determined: How and when?	
Informed, voluntary, limits to confidentiality	
Date of written consent	
Date of verbal consent (clinical confirmation)	
Sources of Information	
Client interview(s) (with structured interview)	
Collateral interview(s)	
Official documentation	
Psychometric testing	
Risk appraisal instruments	
Limitations arising from information sources	
Report Content	
Assessment Context	
Outline of referral source and reason	
Description of evaluation process	
Description of consent process	
Interview impressions	
Psychosocial History	
Family of origin, childhood, adolescence	
Marital/intimate relationships	
Education, employment, and financial	
Leisure	
Substance use/abuse	
Attitudes, associates, and attributions	
Psychological/mental health functioning	
Psychosexual development and behavior (for sexual violence)	

History of Violence and Criminal Behavior	
Offence history	
Current offense	
Institutional behavior (if incarcerated)	
Prior release behavior (if applicable)	
Risk Assessment and Management	
Risk factors	
Actuarial estimates of risk	
Release plans	
Recommendations for managing risk	
Report Distribution	
Date report shared with assessed person, opportunity provided for explanation	
Date corrections/revisions	
Date final report distributed	

FIGURE 6.1. Checklist for risk assessment process.

defensible process, you will be able to defend it through knowledge of the literature. A standardized approach will also serve to increase reliability of measurement and reduce error and the possibility of missing vital information. Finally, a standardized approach allows you to easily respond to questions regarding the process you utilize in your violence risk assessments. It enables you to state with confidence that your approach consists of certain specified procedures (best practices) and will increase your ease of responding to procedural questions, which is particularly relevant when testifying in court regarding your findings and opinions.

Once you have established a standardized approach you must stick to the data (central findings). In concert with Heltzel (2007), keep in mind that your aim is to provide an evaluation that is objective, valid, reliable, and reflects expert neutrality. Practically, you do this by arguing for the data that emerge from the assessment process you employ. Leave aside subjective judgments, and focus on the data. Stay close to the data. It's a good friend. Not only is this good psychological practice, but the courts are putting pressure on experts to focus on the data rather than on "expert opinion" (Hunter et al., 2005). Heilbrun et al. (2007) go a step further and suggest that when the clinician determines that there are substantial barriers to his

Ethics and Consent

Due to the nature and potential outcomes, including loss of liberties, for risk assessments, transparency is of utmost importance. Specifically, your risk assessment must begin with informed consent. As noted in Chapter 1, informed consent is an ethical obligation because you must attain the informed consent of individuals using language that is reasonably understandable to that person or persons (Standard 3.10 of the American Psychological Association, 2002). The informed consent doctrine as it pertains to treatment is clear with regard to informing clients of the benefits and risks of therapeutic procedures (see Meisel, Roth, & Lidz, 1977; Roth, Meisel, & Lidz, 1977); however, the doctrine is less prominent for forensic psychological or psychiatric evaluations (Melton et al., 2007), including risk assessments. Nevertheless, clients must be informed of their rights, even when they elect not to participate in the examination.

Although the doctrine of informed consent is less relevant to the violence risk evaluation process than to treatment situations, it is not irrelevant: informed consent *must* be obtained. Informed consent has three primary elements: adequate disclosure, competency, and voluntariness (Melton et al,. 2007; Stanley & Galietta, 2006). Clients being evaluated for risk of violence must be provided adequate information about the nature and purpose of the evaluation in language that is understandable to them. In other words, you, the examiner, are responsible for disclosing to the offender why you are doing your evaluation, who requested the evaluation, what you will be doing during the evaluation, what you will do with the data you gather, and finally, how the information will be used by the referral source (whether the referral source be a court of law, parole board, or other governing body). We cannot emphasize enough the importance of your ensuring informed consent. It is not sufficient for you to simply provide clients with a written informed consent form. Rather, it is the responsibility of you, the examiner, to ensure that the client has attained sufficient information to allow for competent decision making with regard to his or her participation or refusal to participate in the risk assessment.

Competency to consent is characterized by the client's ability to communicate a choice about his or her participation status, understand relevant assessment-related information, appreciate the nature and purpose of the evaluation and implications of participating or not participating, and manipulate information in a rational manner (Appelbaum & Grisso, 1988). Thus, you, as the examiner, must ensure that clients you evaluate evidence these four standards. You must do this via a documented assessment of the client's competence to consent anytime you suspect a client lacks any one of these four abilities. For example, clients suffering mental illnesses or mental retardation may lead you to question their ability to appreciate the nature and purpose of the evaluation, or to understand the consequences of refusing to participate in the evaluation process; thus, you must assess the client's competency by asking him or her to explain the nature and purpose of the evaluation. Finally, it is your responsibility, to the extent possible, to ensure the client's voluntary participation in the process.

Voluntary participation can be a problem in risk assessments because clients have the right to refuse to participate, but they must be informed of the potential consequences of this decision without being coerced into participating. Voluntariness in risk assessments refers to the clients' utilization of free choice as opposed to responding to third-party influence such as the court or parole board (Melton et al., 2007). You should be particularly sensitive to issues of coercion when completing risk assessments on offenders who are incarcerated, as institutionalization increases powerlessness (see Melton et al., 2007). Incarcerated offenders, for example, may be more inclined to participate against their wishes or reasoned thought simply for fear that the clinician may develop a negative impression of them and therefore detail this impression in subsequent reports to governing bodies responsible for the offender's legal status. Thus, it is incumbent upon you to present clients all options and the consequences of those options when informing them of the nature and purpose of the evaluation. Specifically, you should inform the client of all potential negative consequences for his or her decisions, regardless if he or she is choosing to participate or not. Additionally, it may be beneficial to provide the incarcerated offender time to reflect on his or her options before securing his or her decision. For example, you may inform an offender of the nature and purpose of an evaluation, with all relevant potential consequences, a day or two prior to initiating the evaluation, thus allowing the offender time to reflect upon and consider his or her options (see Stanley & Galietta, 2006).

It is worth reemphasizing that clients have the right to refuse to participate in a risk assessment without prejudice, penalty, or punishment; however, they are still entitled to full disclosure (Conroy, 2003). In other words, you must still provide a complete and thorough explanation of the nature and purpose of the evaluation and explain possible consequences of a refusal to participate as well as consequences for participating. Only then can you ensure that the offender has been fully informed and is prepared and competent to provide informed consent.

In some jurisdictions, a risk assessment would be required and conducted based upon the review of file and collateral sources in the absence of the client's consent and participation. In such cases, we strongly suggest that you refer to this effort as a "risk opinion" or "risk review" and not as a "risk assessment"—a risk assessment includes, at a minimum, all of the elements outlined in this book.

or her impartiality (i.e., he or she feels a desire to advocate for the assessed person), the referred assessment should be declined.

INFORMATION GATHERING

Multimodal Assessment

Generally speaking, information obtained from multiple sources (multimodal assessment) is the preferred method when completing a violence risk assessment. Often, apart from police records or court transcripts that typically describe the crime, little third-party information is available when conducting a violence risk assessment. The exception may be when the individual has been incarcerated in a prison or forensic hospital for a lengthy period of time. File information has been shown to be a rich source of information to allow for the effective scoring of many risk assessment tools, as the retrospective studies reported in Chapter 3 will attest. We submit that third-party information should always be sought to ensure that more objective information is included in the assessment process. Notably, third-party information may subsequently be unavailable, but it should always be sought when conducting violence risk assessments. Although this information is not strictly necessary, it is definitely preferred and will make for a more comprehensive and accurate appraisal and avoid missed information that may later be brought to light as highly relevant. Further, if you do not have the benefit of third-party information, then you should appropriately identify this lack in the evaluation process section of your report (see Chapter 7).

Sources of information may include the results of your semistructured interview, psychometric testing, collateral contacts both personal (family) and professional (e.g., caseworker, psychologist), police reports, prior criminal justice reports, court transcripts, judge's reasons for sentencing, presentence reports, victim impact statements, or prior mental health records (including psychological tests and actuarial measures).

The Semistructured Interview

The semistructured interview is sometimes referred to as an *aide memoire* (a device that serves to aid memory). It simply refers to an interview document that contains a list of questions covering a variety of areas of relevance to the assessment at hand. Aide memoire will differ depending on the outcome of interest. It would be possible to fashion one that would cover different types of violence, but experience has shown that the types of questions one would ask when conducting an assessment for sexual recidivism would be quite different than what would be used to assess a client for domestic violence. The point here is simply to ensure that you have one. Developing the aide memoire will take some time, but the exercise of developing the questions that you will need to cover all of the areas of interest will be invaluable. We typically encourage those who are new to violence assessment to consult colleagues for samples of their aide memoire as a place to start. Structure your interview to include both open-ended questions that will give you a better sense of the client's interpersonal characteristics as well as some yes/no questions to determine if an area is in need of further exploration. The semistructured aspect simply means that there are certain questions that you will ask with plenty of room for follow-up questions for clarification. Using such interviewing skills as paraphrasing, probes, continuation prompts, and reflection will result in greater ease in gathering the information and contribute to the flow of the interview. This semistructured style will ensure that you ask questions relevant to the risk factors for the outcome, that is, you will include risk factors in general as well as those specifically needed to score risk appraisal instruments.

A helpful feature that you can build into an aide memoire is the specific questions that you need answered in order to score the risk appraisal instrument you are using. As an example, we have developed our own aide memoire which have in the margin the item number from the instrument of interest. For instance, if we utilized the LSI-R, then beside the questions that asked the client about his or her level of education we would place the corresponding LSI-R item numbers that the answers assist in scoring. In doing so we ensure that we ask sufficient questions to score the risk appraisal instruments relevant to the outcome. In addition to questions relevant to the scoring of risk appraisal instruments, the issue of consent should be included in your semistructured interview. We routinely note, at beginning of the document, that the process of the assessment was discussed with the client and that the issues of consent were reviewed with them. We further note whether we were satisfied that those issues were understood and consent was granted. Also, it is possible to leave space on the aide memoire where brief notations can be made regarding third-party documentation that either support or contradict the client's assertions. Your semistructured interview document then becomes a key to integrating the various sources of information around the risk factors. Keep in mind that the aide memoire is a part of the client's file which may be subpoenaed to court during disclosure. With this in mind, be careful what you *doodle* in the margins or what *vernacular* language you may use to describe the client.

Psychometric Questionnaires

Clinicians will often use psychometric questionnaires as part of their assessment process. We use the term *psychometric instrument* to refer to paper-and-pencil or computer-administered self-report questionnaires that are scored and compared to a normative group. Strictly speaking, psychometric instruments are not necessary to conduct an assessment of violence risk. However, psychometric tests can assist the clinician in a number of helpful ways. As in any clinical assessment, psychometric instruments can cover a broad array of psychopathology or personality domains and provide the clinician with a picture of how the individual compares with the normative groups. These test results are hypotheses that should be explored in the interview before drawing any conclusions. We have found that psychometric testing can provide a useful source of information in the multimodal approach to risk appraisal. Specifically, psychometric instruments can inform on certain risk factors such as anger, antisocial attitudes, and antisocial associates. Among sex offenders, psychometric instruments may inform on attitudes, cognitive distortions, and sexual deviance. Among spousal assaulters psychometric instruments can inform on attitudes toward women and attitudes toward violence. Additionally, psychometric instruments can provide information on symptoms of mental illness as well as data about personality character-istics and interpersonal style.

Unless specifically designed to do so, psychometric instruments should *never* be used to estimate likelihood to reoffend. There are occasions where clinicians have become very familiar with specific psychometric tools and have placed their unwarranted faith in those instruments while ignoring much more accurate estimates provided by risk appraisal instruments. You will recall in the opening chapter to this book our discussion of the reliance of clinicians on instruments such as the MMPI, which have been clearly shown to be inferior predictors of violence. An example of the misuse of a psychometric instrument was provided by a colleague who is an expert in sexual offender assessment and treatment. A risk assessment report con-tained the results of the MCMI-III which apparently indicated that the cli-ent presented with symptoms of schizoid personality traits with some self-defeating features. Based on the results of the MCMI-III and consultations with others, the psychologist made the following statement: "It should be noted that Mr. Client's current psychological status pooled with his histori-cal pattern of criminality portended an extremely high risk, if not approach-ing certainty, for criminal recidivism if he were to be released to the commu-nity." Our colleague went on to note that when she assessed this same client, the client received a score of 2 on the Static-99, which is associated with recidivism rates for sexual reoffending of 9% over 5 years and 13% over 10 years, and for violent (including sexual) reoffense of 17% over 5 years and 25% over 10 years. In our opinion, the use of measures of personality functioning and psychopathology (e.g., MMPI, MCMI, PAI) and clinical judgment to draw such a conclusion is indefensible and does not meet mini-mum standards of practice. We do not know the client nor the professional who made the judgment but this is an example where a professional would have no empirical defense for making such a statement, is providing a dis-service to the populations served (including both the referral source and the offender) as well as the profession, and is opening him- or herself up to censure if a complaint was ever lodged.

When using psychometric instruments, we recommend that you score and review the results and any critical items in a timely manner after the cli-ent has completed the test instrument(s). Why? Because you are responsible for any information that you have in your possession even if it has not been scored. If, for example, a client endorses items suggesting a risk for self-harm on an instrument such as the PAI and makes a suicide attempt while the instrument has sat unscored in your inbox for several weeks, you may be liable since you had information that could have indicated that the client was at risk and warranted a referral to rule out this possibility. This liability may still be present even if the client did not report those thoughts or feelings during the interview. We advocate that you arrange for the psychometric test results to be scored soon after completion and reviewed for indicators of suicide, self-harm, or harm to others. Endorsed indicators should result in a referral (more likely if the person is institutionalized) or personal follow-up.

Another issue is the timing of psychometric testing. Some clinicians prefer to interview the client and then determine the "appropriate" tests to be administered, while others want to have the psychometric instruments completed prior to the interview in order to appropriately test hypotheses raised by the psychometric results. We would advocate for the latter insofar as violence risk assessment should be a very standardized process as we have already discussed: therefore you should have already determined in advance the tests that you would use to assess the referral question. There may be occasions when specific issues arise that may be of relevance to the case but were not foreseen and follow up testing may be indicated, but these should be the exception not the rule. Completing psychometric instruments first avoids the problem of having to follow-up with inconsistencies between the psychometric test results and your interview findings.

REPORTING THE FINDINGS

Webster, Hucker, and Bloom (2002) suggest that a risk assessment needs to meet five criteria. First, it should demonstrate an understanding of the legal context within which the information will be considered and then provide information that is legally relevant. Second, the assessment must be conducted and reported in an evidence-based and scientific manner. Specifically, every reasonable effort should be made to gather information, state limitations of knowledge, and report the findings in a logical and concise format. Third, a risk assessment should contain a statement of risk which may include circumstances that may alter risk, identify potential victims, and express a likely time frame with a probability of occurrence. Fourth, the report should suggest how the risk of the individual would be best managed. Fifth, and this is more of a prospective suggestion, examiners should compare the individual case with data from statistically driven studies.

Other experts in the field have made a number of suggestions for improving risk assessment reports (Heilbrun, Dvoskin, et al., 1999). These include the use of plain language in reports so that the lay consumer can easily understand what is reported. The purpose of the assessment should be clearly stated and the process undertaken well described. Multiple sources of information should be employed, with observations made regarding discrepancies. The assessment report should summarize the information from which opinions and recommendations will be drawn. Risk should be related to time, specifically, what level of risk over what time period. Estimates of risk should be based upon actuarial data whenever possible. In addition, recommendations should be made for the appropriate intervention to address the risk factors and strategies to manage risk should also be articulated.

We would like to reinforce in particular the use of plain language within forensic reports. As a general guideline, if your word processor does not recognize the word or your dictionary does not contain the word, then use another word or define and explain the term. For example, when reading a recent risk assessment we encountered terms like *autogynephilia* (a man's sexual disorder that results in his arousal at the thought of having a woman's body, usually relating to sex organs) and *egodystonic* (thoughts and behaviors that are not consistent with the person's self-image), which were not defined or explained for the reader and would leave some experienced clinicians scrambling for a clinical thesaurus. We urge you to consider your audience and remember that the consumer of your assessment is a professional (e.g., judge, lawyer, probation officer, prison official) like yourself whose time is valuable. Good report writers will not force their readers to search for the meanings of words that are uncommon in general language (i.e., professional jargon) and specific to a particular field of study. Some areas particularly fraught with this tendency are the reporting of projective tests, the communication of certain diagnoses, and the assessment of sexual paraphilias (unusual sexual activity; DSM-IV-TR [American Psychiatric Association, 2000]). (*Note: paraphilias* is not recognized by most word processors and is not easily found in standard dictionaries.)

Chapter 7 outlines in more detail a suggested risk assessment report format. Before discussing the format in detail, we wish to note some general principles that should be considered. Clinicians vary with regard to their style of report writing. For example, one of us (RM) relies on a traditional clinical report format modified to present information relevant to violence risk assessment. Two of us, on the other hand, recommend telling a story about the individual rather than writing a typical clinical report. A story is more easily understood and the client's behavior is placed within the context of his or her own personal history and others' behavior (risk appraisal and estimates). How you ultimately choose to write a risk assessment is a matter of personal style and it will influence the *order* of the report's content; however, your knowledge and due diligence will guarantee that the content itself will be consistent. Therefore, while the presentation may change, the content should differ little between individuals.

Another advantage of telling a story is that an explanation of the client's behavior can be more readily communicated. Whereas many referral sources simply request an assessment of risk, we have observed that in contentious cases where decisions are being made about release or reduction in security, decision makers are also seeking an understanding of why the person committed the act in the first place. This is particularly true in cases where the client has a limited history of antisocial behavior yet has acted in a very violent manner. It is our observation that decision makers appreciate having a fuller understanding of why the offense occurred.

When telling the story, be sure to correctly attribute the various sources of information. We have broken this out into four types of information: source information (i.e., what the client or others have told you), facts, assumptions, and opinions. When the source of information is from the client, ensure the use of terms such as "Mr. Client reported (recalled, informed, indicated, etc.) that he was physically abused by his father" as opposed to "Mr. Client was abused by his father." If you have independent information from other sources such as child welfare services that abuse definitely took place, then you could report, "Mr. Client reported that he was physically abused by his father and this is supported by information from child protective services." What you want to avoid is reporting what the client said as fact. Facts will be determined by the judicial or quasi-judicial system for which the report is being prepared. If information you receive from other sources can be verified independently as having occurred, then it may be stated as fact and it is acceptable to do so: "Mr. Client was convicted of assault causing bodily harm." Sometimes there is a collection of information from which you may draw a conclusion or make an assumption. Continuing with the same example of childhood abuse, if the client reported numerous points of information indicating abuse, parental violence, and general dysfunction in the home, you might conclude, "Taken together, it would appear that Mr. Client had a difficult start in life and experienced considerable abuse, neglect, and poor role modeling within his family of origin." Finally, when you offer a professional opinion, then you need to be explicit that it is your opinion and recapitulate the facts upon which the opinion is based.

Depending on the setting in which you are assessing, one of the first persons to read the report is the client (the assessed person). Where possible in practice, we offer the client an opportunity to read the report. He or she is given a pencil to circle any "errors of fact," for example, if mistakes may have been made in terms of dates and times or personal historical information. We also advise the client in advance that we are open to correcting any historical inaccuracies but the conclusions are our professional judgment for which we have been retained. Admittedly, there are only a few occasions that require corrections but by involving the client we continue our commitment to transparency in the risk assessment process. Other benefits include both the client and other parties understanding your commitment to accuracy (you would not want someone getting even small things wrong about the details of your life) and we reduce error in the final report to avoid errors coming to light in court where small inaccuracies can be used by opposing counsel to challenge the overall accuracy of the assessment. Also, by advising the client he or she will have this opportunity, you may reduce the adversarial nature of the assessment context.

Focusing on the Referral Question

When writing a violence risk assessment, keep the focus on the referral question, to the exclusion of other issues. The content of the assessment should only include information that is going to inform the answer to the question. This may mean a change for some people more than others depending upon the style of writing in which they have been trained. Focusing on the question can mean making both small and large changes to content. For example, we had a colleague who introduced the client in an assessment thus: "Black, slight-built male." This descriptive style of presenting race, physical attributes, and gender no doubt came out of the clinician's clinical training of years ago. However, the inmate complained that his being black was not an issue; his complaint was upheld following institutional review. The rationale for the legal opinion was "irrelevant information should not be included and that as a matter of style, it would be better not to include irrelevant references that obviously have offended people." However, should tests have been utilized that required different cultural norms according to race, then including a description of race would be relevant, but this too must be explained in order that the information can be deemed relevant.

In another example of irrelevant information the following quote was taken from an assessment at an intake unit for the purpose of identifying risk factors and suggesting intervention priorities. Using a projective test the clinician concluded the following in regards to the client: "Object relations are at a primitive level with the offender fixated in a dyadic struggle between enmeshment which he fears would totally obliterate his nascent identity and total isolation which is equated with traumatic abandonment. Primary preoccupations over separation issues and anxiety as related to the sense of self is embattled." Apart from a lay consumer of the report being at a total loss to understand the content, we remain perplexed as to how this identifies risk factors and appropriate treatment or programing options. The need to communicate useful information is of paramount importance because to do otherwise suggests to consumers that we have nothing of value to add.

You will recall from an earlier paragraph in this chapter our account of the "near certainty" prediction based upon the MCMI-III and clinical judgment. That same assessment also included the following information regarding diagnoses: "Axis 1: Gerontophilia; Cocaine Abuse, In a Controlled Environment; History of Polysubstance Dependence; Male Erectile Disorder by Patient Self-report. Axis II: Psychopathic Personality Disorder with Prominent Schizoid Features and Pseudologia Phantastica. Axis III: Diabetes Mellitus, Hep C." For some professionals it is a practice to diagnose individuals on whom routine assessments are conducted but a violence risk assessment is not a routine clinical evaluation. In keeping with the principle of providing information that is only relevant to the referral question, it would be inappropriate to refer to the client's erectile disorder unless it was germane to the assessment of risk. As we have already indicated to comment on a diagnosis of psychopathic personality disorder without using one of the PCL instruments is professionally skating on very thin ice indeed, not to mention that psychopathic personality was not recognized by the DSM-IV. One of us (RM) discovered that including unrelated diagnosis can be used to extend an offender's sanction. For example, in a routine forensic assessment a diagnosis unrelated to the psycholegal issue was used in the punishment phase to increase the offender's sentencing. Recognizing the disservice this provided to the offender specifically and the criminal justice system more broadly, we have taken to advocating that only those diagnoses directly relevant to the question at hand (e.g., Is this individual a risk for violence?) be included in the report. In fact, to make this explicitly clear, one of us (RM) has taken to including a diagnostic section that explicitly states that the listed diagnoses are limited to those psychiatric diagnoses directly relevant to the risk appraisal (i.e., "The following DSM-IV-TR diagnoses are relevant to the issue of this client's violence risk appraisal").

A clear and transparent approach to the process of violence risk assessment reflects that you have thought through the central issues and have structured the evaluation in such a way that it will cover all of the central and important issues systematically. Considerable knowledge and effort will be necessary for you to put into place an effective process, but once you have done that, "tweaking" your process later based upon new information will generally require a modest effort. Get the process right the first time.

To this point we have covered a lot of ground to prepare you for the final effort, which is the report. In the next chapter we examine writing the report. This is the point where your knowledge of violence risk assessment and process integrate to tell the story of the individual and explain how and why he or she has arrived at this point and what risk he or she poses to society.

CHAPTER 7

■   ■   ■

TELLING THE STORY

An Outline for the Report

As we suggested in Chapter 4 and elsewhere, communicating violence risk estimates should not happen only in the report paragraphs that specifically address actuarial estimates. Conveying risk estimates alone is insufficient; you need to place them in the context of a story that explains them (Dawes, 1999; Schwalbe, 2004). The risk assessment report is that story. Robyn Dawes (1999) drew from research into the process of jury decision making to support this contention that information is believed when it appears within the context of a good story. Further, Dawes argues that for issues such as base rates, a story that suggests causality makes them relevant, leading to the conclusion that "we do not appreciate probability without the story" (p. 39). Chapter 6 laid out the risk assessment process. In this chapter we cover in considerable detail the writing of the report. We will reiterate one important point from Chapter 6: personal style will dictate how a report is structured, but due diligence will determine its content. The style proposed here is structured to tell the individual's story:

Why is he or she here? (Assessment Context)
Where did he or she come from? (Psychosocial Background)
What has he or she done? (History of Violence and Criminal Behavior)
What can be done about it? (Risk Assessment and Risk Management)

We are not suggesting that this is the only structure a report should take, but clinicians have routinely asked us for report samples to help them in practice, so we have included this as one possible outline to consider. It is not essential that you employ the same headings and titles, but you should cover the same content. A sample report following this outline is provided in the Appendix.

Another difference that we take in structuring a report that will differ considerably from more typical clinical assessments is the manner in which we integrate the results of psychometric testing. Traditionally, clinical reports have a separate section where psychometric tests are reported and interpreted. We view the psychometric test as another source of information that should be woven into the report where the content is being addressed. For example, we would interpret psychometric measures of psychopathology (e.g., PAI, MMPI) in the section on the individual's psychological and mental health functioning. We may also refer to the same psychometric instruments a second time if those instruments spoke to issues of interpersonal style which may inform a supervision strategy. It is our opinion that this spares the reader, who is often a lay consumer of the report, the task of trying to integrate psychometric tests reported in one section with information reported in another section and serves to promote a more fluid structure to the report.

ASSESSMENT CONTEXT

The Assessment Context lays out for the reader your understanding of the who, what, where, why, and how of the assessment. It is essential that your assessment be set within the appropriate context and that you communicate your understood role in and method for conducting the assessment. We have broken this section into the referral, the evaluation process (which includes the psychometric instruments and risk appraisal instruments utilized and the sources of information), the consent process, and general interview impressions.

Referral

In the referral section you will want to ensure that you identify the source of the referral and why. Specifically you would identify who retained your services. This will usually be legal counsel or it may be an institutional/system requirement if the client is in custody. If the client has been convicted for an offense, then the offense(s) and disposition should be delineated. You should then identify why you were asked to conduct the assessment. Is it part of an institutional review to determine parole suitability or placement at a lower security forensic institution or is the assessment part of a sentencing process? Then make clear what it is you intend to accomplish. That is to say, you need to identify what your assessment will produce. Specifically, what value-added information will your assessment have that answers the referral question? Among the many assessment outcomes could be determining the risk the client poses for future violence, developing interventions to manage the risk of violence, or identifying treatment priorities.

> Mr. Client is a 32-year-old male with a history of criminal and violent offending. He is currently serving a sentence of 5 years for the offenses of Aggravated Assault and Failure to Comply with a Probation Order. The referral for this assessment was made by D. B., parole officer at XYZ Institution, for the purpose of determining his suitability for release. The present report will identify risk factors for future criminal and violent behavior, assess Mr. Client's risk to re-offend, and make recommendations on how to best intervene and manage that risk.

Evaluation Process

In this section you will report how you conducted your assessment. You should be specific in detailing the process you undertook. This should at the very least include an interview(s) and a review of collateral information; in most cases it will also include psychometric tests. When describing the process, be specific as to dates and length of time. Be aware that this reporting is part of the transparency of the assessment process. You should also be aware that specific reporting can insulate you from criticism. For example, if one of the parties to the process, whether it is the client, his or her representative, or an opposing party complains that you arrived at your conclusions without sufficient time spent on the case, you will have documented information to the contrary. This will also work against you if you attempted short-cuts. For example, if you scored the VRAG as part of your assessment, was there sufficient documented time to determine a PCL-R score (although the CATS substitute takes less time) and diagnose or rule out schizophrenia and personality disorder which are all components of the VRAG? Times, places for interviews, and testing should be reported. If you used the services of an unlicensed practitioner for aspects of the assessment process such as psychometric test administration, this information should also be included. Then specify that he or she was trained and his or her participation was within generally accepted practices (make sure it is). Also included here is an outline of the information that you considered. For example, you would include a list of all of the documents (court documents or file information), collateral sources (interviews with other professionals or family, review of medical records), psychometric tests used, and risk appraisal instruments employed that you considered when forming your opinion.

The question of how specific to be when identifying documents or files read in the conducting of an assessment has often been posed. That is, does one refer to having reviewed a file or to each specific report in the file? This question often occurs in cases where there is a lot of documentation that has accumulated over time. In answering this question we would first refer you back to your own licensing body because their requirements may differ. We have seen reports that have simply listed the "files reviewed" with no specificity as to the documents or reports read—this is not an acceptable practice. At the other end of the spectrum we have seen reports with pages listing every document read whether it appeared relevant or otherwise. Depending on the record-keeping requirements of different facilities, some files may be burdened with many notes and records that have no relevance to your assessment; documenting these when they have no bearing on the assessment is not helpful. Our recommendation is that in instances where there is a lot of documentation you should report the files you had access to and then report all of the documents that you *actually* considered as part of the assessment process. Be very sure that if you used a piece of information that was present (you identified an institutional charge in a document) or absent (you could not find an institutional charge in the file) in your assessment, that you identify specifically what you considered and how you determined the information. This may appear laborious but it is essential to transparency and will spare you many woes in contentious cases.

> This assessment is based on clinical interviews with Mr. Client at the XYZ Institution on February 14, 20XX, from 2:00 P.M. to 4:00 P.M. and on February 15, 20XX, from 9:00 A.M. to 10:30 A.M. Additionally, psychological testing (as outlined below) was completed by Mr. Client on February 7, 20XX. The case management files, psychology file, and medical records were made available to me and the relevant documents considered in this assessment are listed below. Based on the clinical interview and information reviewed, the following risk appraisal instruments were scored: the Sex Offender Risk Appraisal Guide (estimate of violence risk) and the Static-99 (estimate of risk for sexual reoffending).

Consent

Obtaining and reporting informed consent is of paramount importance in an assessment process (and may be statutorily required). Often times consent may be *initiated* through a signed form. This may occur at times through the referral agent if that agent is legal counsel. However, it is essential that you remember that *a signed consent form is not informed consent*. Informed consent is the clinician's determination that the client is capable of making informed consent: he or she understands all of the aspects of the assessment process which includes but is not limited to limits of confidentiality, right to withdraw, and parties to whom the assessment will be released; and to the extent possible, voluntarily agrees to participate in the assessment process. This determination can only occur when the clinician takes the time to review the specific issues contained in the consent form with the client and determines that the client understands and gives informed consent. The process of obtaining informed consent should be explicitly documented. You should be aware that delegating the process of informed consent is not recommended because it is the licensed professional who must attest that the individual met all of the requirements of informed consent including having the capacity to give informed consent.

> Mr. Client reviewed my consent form with his legal counsel which outlined the nature of the assessment process, the limits of confidentiality, the parties to whom the report would be provided, and mandatory reporting requirements, and his voluntary participation in the process. Mr. Client signed the form indicating his consent on February 5, 20XX. Prior to our clinical interview of February 14th, 20XX, I reviewed the content of the consent form with Mr. Client and I was satisfied that he was competent to give consent, that he understood the content and issues contained in the consent form, and that he gave his informed consent to proceed with the assessment process.

Interview Impressions

The interview impression section reports what is quite typical in most clinical reports with which you will be familiar. Here you would report the client's willingness to engage in the interview process, his or her manner of responding, and how forthcoming he or she was with information. You would report how the client tended to answer questions in terms of brevity or comprehensiveness. Report if he or she refused to respond, avoided, or evaded answering certain questions. You would identify if he or she attempted to control the interview, if he or she could remain goal-directed, or if he or she needed to be redirected to topics of discussion. You would also report the client's insight into his or her own behavior, whether he or she expressed remorse, and his or her affective presentation. This would include observations of body language, expressed anger, hostility, or suspiciousness. It is important to also report positive presentations and cooperation provided by the client. Any observations regarding symptoms of mental illness, mood disturbance, or anxiety should also be noted.

PSYCHOSOCIAL BACKGROUND

The purpose of this section is to set the client within the context of his or her personal history. At its essence we answer three questions: Who is the client, where did the client come from, and how did the client get here? It is important that the consumer of the assessment understand that behavior does not happen within a vacuum and that individuals arrive at a behavior pattern from different origins. A detailed personal history also helps to answer or explain how the individual has come to this point in his or her life and how or why he or she has acted as he or she has. Also, it provides the client with an indication that he or she has been heard and understood. He or she may not agree with your ultimate determination of risk, but he or she will at least understand that you took the time to be comprehensive and report both the positive and negative aspects of his or her background. We can never forget that in the midst of an adversarial system there is a person at the center of the decision and we have ethical and moral obligations to him or her.

Another important point to remember is that the information we draw upon to assess the risk for violence should be contained in this section and in the Offense History section of the report. For example, if you use the LSI-R as your estimate of violence risk, you should ensure that the domains and questions covered by the LSI-R are reported in the Psychosocial History section. Though not necessarily item by item, this section should contain enough information that another professional would be able to determine how and why you arrived at your scores on your risk instruments simply by reading the assessment. We have divided this section into family of origin, childhood, and adolescence; education, employment, and financial history; substance abuse/dependence; marital/intimate relationships; associates, attitudes, and attributions; and psychological/mental health functioning. In instances where the question of sexual behavior is central to the assessment, such as cases where the issues are sexual violence or there is evidence of sexual paraphilas, then we would recommend adding a further section on psychosexual development. In cases where the issue of sexual conduct is not central, then basic sexual developmental information could be reported under the first heading.

Family of Origin, Childhood, and Adolescence

Within this section you want to describe the parents and siblings, preadolescent years (birth to 12 years), and adolescent years (13–18 years), with a focus on issues and facts of relevance to violence or criminal offending. This format first describes the client's developmental environment and then specifically identifies his or her behavior patterns within that environment.

This would include issues of parental involvement (biological or adoptive parents), family stability (parental relationship), and parental modeling of behavior both prosocial (stable employment, education, financially responsible) and antisocial. Document any parental and sibling involvement in violent, criminal, or antisocial behavior, drug and/or alcohol abuse, and mental health issues. Report any disruption in the family such as marital breakdowns, the involvement of child protective services, or turnover in parental figures. Identify type and frequency of parental discipline, looking for evidence of abuse as well as any violence in the home that the client may have been subject to or witnessed. These issues speak to the behavior learned through observation and experience in the family of origin.

When considering child and adolescent behavior, identify the onset, frequency, and severity of antisocial behavior whether in childhood or adolescence. Issues in childhood and adolescence would also include school performance, grade level completed, drug and/or alcohol abuse, onset of sexual activity, social functioning and associates whether antisocial or prosocial, adult/parental supervision, criminal charges, and admissions to custody. Determine if the client was a bully or the victim of bullying. Report on police contacts, peers, and absences from home without permission. Recall that this information is also necessary to score a number of risk instruments such as the VRAG, the SORAG, and the LSI-R.

Education, Employment, and Financial History

Education, employment, and financial problems are risk factors for criminal behavior and violence. Reporting on the client's educational background can inform on his or her behavior during childhood and adolescence, his or her ability to interact with authority figures, and his or her ability to secure and maintain self-supporting employment. You want to determine the client's attendance (truancy), interaction with teachers, grades obtained, placement in special education, failure of individual courses or grades, diagnoses if any of a learning disability, as well as current commitment to education to further employment opportunities. In terms of employment background, you should identify the number and types of jobs performed (what specifically did he or she do and for how long), skills acquired, and the reasons why he or she left those jobs (e.g., fired, bored, imprisoned, or for a better paying job). If there were periods of unemployment, determine what was going on and how he or she was supported. Both education and employment history lead nicely in to the client's financial history. This would include if he or she has been self-supporting or has relied on social assistance, disability benefits, family, or crime to provide financial support. You want to determine if he or she has a bank account, savings, or outstanding debts. The information here needs to be sufficient to describe the client's ability to secure and manage financial resources, as financial stressors may precipitate criminal or violent behavior.

Marital/Intimate Relationships

Following a comprehensive assessment of the client's formative and adolescent years the next section covers the issue of marital/intimate and adult family relationships. Record here the number of sexual partners, number of committed relationships, the level of commitment, and practical support of spouse and children. If there have been multiple live-in partners, determine why the relationships ended, and specifically what the issues were and who initiated the separation. Some individuals will verbalize commitment to family and children, but when asked about specifics such as financial support and faithfulness they can provide little evidence to support their assertion.

You will also want to probe the nature of the relationships. You want to determine if those relationships were conflictual, how problems were resolved, how long a relationship lasted, whether there were separations during the relationship, and whether there was any interpersonal violence. Be sure when you ask questions about potential partner violence that you use terms other than "violence" when exploring the possibility. You want to determine the nature and frequency of conflicts (yelling, swearing, etc.). You may ask if the partner ever pushed the client or threw something at the client and then follow up with "Did you ever throw something at your partner or push your partner?" More emphasis will be placed upon this section if one of the referral questions is the risk for spousal/partner violence as the answers will provide information necessary for scoring the risk appraisal instruments.

Substance Use/Abuse

Most clinicians will be familiar with assessing and reporting a history of drug and/or alcohol abuse. This will obviously include onset, severity, whether it is abuse or dependence, whether patterns of use are associated with environmental stressors, and whether the abuse is sporadic or chronic. In addition to the typical review it will be important to determine how drug and/or alcohol abuse relates to the behavior in question. In other words, does the individual act violently only when under the influence of alcohol or illicit substances or are there indications that aggression and violence occur when not using or when experiencing withdrawal? The relationship between substance abuse and violence is quite evident overall; however, in practice some individuals use with such frequency that it is difficult to judge what they would be like if they were sober for any length of time. This also compounds the assessment of other risk factors (such as mental illness, for which we recommend 3 months of sobriety before conducting a diagnostic assessment).

Attitudes, Associates, and Attributions

Attitudes and associates are among the best predictors of criminal behavior (Gendreau et al., 1996). You clearly want to indicate if the client endorses antisocial attitudes and maintains a network of antisocial friends and acquaintances. You would also identify the client's social support systems and any positive people who have influence and regular contact with him or her. Attributions speak to the issue of insight into behavior by identifying to what the client attributes his or her actions. For example, does the client blame the victim ("she provoked me"), does he or she blame alcohol or drugs ("I was stoned at the time"), or does he or she blame society ("I tried to get social assistance but they denied me")? It is important that insofar as attributions inform insight they are not a risk factor; however, attributions may inform on issues of treatment readiness or the integration of treatment benefits. For example, if a sex offender still continues to blame the victim following treatment, the issue of treatment integration needs to be raised. This section is one that provides an opportunity to integrate interview findings with the results of psychometric instruments. Common instruments for the assessment of antisocial cognitions and associates include the Psychological Inventory of Criminal Thinking Styles (PICTS; Walters & White, 1989), the Criminal Sentiments Scale—Modified (CSS-M; Simourd, 1997), and the Measure of Criminal Attitudes and Associates (MCAA: Mills, Kroner, & Hemmati, 2004). You can then incorporate findings from these psychometric measures with your interview findings. For example:

> At points during the interview Mr. Client rationalized his antisocial behavior and expressed an attitude that condoned criminal behavior in certain circumstances. As an example he said that he had always been taught to solve his problems by violence and suggested that sometimes stealing is necessary for survival. A psychometric evaluation of Mr. Client's criminal attitudes and associates was undertaken using the Measures of Criminal Attitudes and Associates (MCAA; Mills & Kroner, 1999). The results indicate that Mr. Client endorses criminal attitudes, specifically attitudes toward violence, antisocial entitlement, and antisocial intent, that exceed those of the average offender in the normative study group. Mr. Client also identified two individuals with whom he spends time who have a history of criminal behavior.

For another example of how psychometric findings of attitudes can be incorporated into a report see the Attitudes, Associates, and Attributions section of the sample report in the Appendix.

Leisure

Leisure activities are an often overlooked but are an important predictor of criminal and violent behavior (Zamble & Quinsey, 1997). During a treatment group that focuses on changing the antisocial associates of offenders, Mills and Kroner (2006c) conduct an exercise to show offenders the amount of spare time they will potentially have available even if they are working full time. Allocating 10 hours for 5 days to work (includes travel), 3 hours per day for personal care (meals, grooming, etc.), 2 hours per day for chores and errands (shopping, dishes, laundry), and 8 hours each day for sleep leaves a total of 27 hours of unstructured time each week. It is not difficult to see the potential problem this free time poses for individuals who have a history of impulsive behavior, substance abuse, and antisocial associates *even if* they have a full-time job. Thus, you will want to report on hobbies, sports activities, family ties, or time with a faith community. Identify leisure activities that are structured, productive, and with prosocial individuals versus leisure time that is unstructured, used in risky pursuits, nonproductive, and includes antisocial peers to guide your recommended risk management strategies.

Psychological/Mental Health Functioning

Historical and current psychological functioning are important indicators of violence risk. This section reports specifically on current and prior mental health diagnoses as well as any identified personality disorder. Any prior admissions or contact with mental health professionals and related treatment or hospitalizations should be reported and whether these were voluntary or involuntary. Report how long the client was hospitalized or treated, any diagnoses, and medication prescribed as they relate to risk or risk management issues. Psychometric instruments (e.g., PAI, MMPI) would be interpreted in this section as they inform on psychopathology (e.g., impulsivity, anger, depression, anxiety) as well as personality functioning (interpersonal style, self-concept, etc.). If you have chosen to score the PCL-R, you will want to record the associated personality characteristics in this section (empathy, callousness, etc.). Also, if assessed, the client's cognitive or memory functioning would be reported here. Medical information is included by some; however, in keeping with the underlying issue of parsimony and focusing on the referral question, we recommend not including that type of information unless it is relevant to the assessment or management of the risk for violence.

As a general principle we have indicated that only information relevant to the assessment question should be included in violence risk assessments. However, given that suicide attempts are related to mental health issues, that many individuals assessed for violence are institutionalized, and that suicide risk is higher among offenders and that suicide is an important custodial issue (Hayes, 1995), we would suggest that a review of suicide/self-harm history and a brief review of current risk factors—including determining if suicidal ideation is present—should be included as a part of the violence risk assessment.

> Mr. Client reported that he has attempted suicide on one occasion which was shortly before his arrest. He informed me that he impulsively consumed a bottle of pain relievers, which made him quite nauseated. Even as he acted he was uncertain of the lethality of his actions and expressed some ambivalence to dying, saying he just did not want to face the charges. He reported during the interview that he was quite depressed and hopeless at the time but it was a single incident and he has not had subsequent thoughts of hurting himself. He indicated that he was overwhelmed by the stress of the moment and acted rashly. Prior to our interview, Mr. Client completed the XYZ instrument and measures of depression and hopelessness were within normal limits and his presentation today was consistent with those results. As noted above, Mr. Client has no history of mental illness, mood disturbance, or personality disorder. He expressed a strong religious prohibition against suicide. Collectively, these findings indicate that Mr. Client does not present as currently at risk for suicide or self-harm.

Psychosexual Development and Behavior

As noted previously, if sexual behavior appears as an issue in the case, whether due to a charge or conviction or whether unusual sexual activities or overtones are present without charges, then a separate section on sexual development and behavior is warranted. Within this section you will need to provide details regarding the onset of sexual behavior, the age-appropriateness of partners, sexual orientation, and any particulars of the development of sexual knowledge. The number and types (short term, casual, or long term) of sexual relationships the client has engaged in should be included. Attempt to determine if sexual relationships were consensual or coerced. "Coerced" does not necessarily mean the use of threats or violence, but may include insistence when the partner said no to sexual relations, or when the partner was intoxicated to the point of not being fully aware of sexual behavior, or if the partner may not have been otherwise competent (a severely cognitively limited individual). Report any use of pornography, onset, frequency, source, and type (adult male or female, child, violence or bondage depicted), as well as use of prostitutes. You will need to report masturbatory behavior and the type of fantasy associated with the behavior. Ensure you report any atypical sexual behaviors such as sadomasochism, voyeurism, incest, exhibitionism, frotterism, bestiality, or group sex. It is also recommended that you provide the results of phallometric testing if that is available.

HISTORY OF VIOLENCE AND CRIMINAL BEHAVIOR
Offense History

When reviewing the client's offense history you want to ensure that you include all of the offense convictions and not simply those that relate to violence. Recall from our previous discussion that criminal *nonviolent* behavior is a risk factor for violence and many instruments include this history directly into the estimates of risk. You will have already reported the onset of more general antisocial behavior in the Psychosocial History section but in this section you want to focus on the client's criminal behavior. Be sure to include the age of onset of criminal behavior, as well as the onset of violent behavior. This would include any criminal behavior committed as a juvenile. Report the severity and frequency of criminal and violent behavior. You will want to consider the client's persistence in criminal behavior as well as any meaningful breaks from criminal behavior. These breaks should be examined to determine what was occurring in his or her life at the time that seemed to keep him or her from reoffending. Also look for patterns, antecedents, and correlates of violent and criminal behavior. In the interview process you will likely get a sense of how the client views his or her behavior, the level of insight into why he or she acts violently, and what if anything he or she believes he or she needs to do to change.

Current Offense

With respect to the current offense, ensure that you have all of the specifics of the client's actions as they have been reported in official documents. Be sure to compare the client's version with the official version and ask for clarifications on any discrepancies. Seek to understand the client's level of admission to and responsibility for the offense. Place the current offense within the client's behavioral or criminal history and report any patterns, antecedents, and correlates to the current offense. Look for specific insight into the current offense and determine if there is anything significantly different from the current offense and its precipitators and past behavior patterns.

Institutional Behavior

Institutional behavior has been found by some to be a risk factor for reoffending, but is reflected in some but not all risk assessment instruments

(Brown et al., 2009; Nugent, 2000). This may not be relevant to all cases if the client is not incarcerated (e.g., pending a trial). However, where available, information regarding misconduct and aggression within the institution should be reviewed with the client and documented. This behavior should be examined within the context of previous community behavior, looking for any continuance of patterns, antecedents, or correlates.

Prior Release Behavior

Prior release behavior is related to criminal recidivism, in particular new crimes and failures to comply with probation/parole conditions. Even in cases where the client has not been previously incarcerated, he or she may be on some form of court-ordered conditional release pending completion of trial proceedings and his or her behavior during this time frame is relevant.

RISK ASSESSMENT AND RISK MANAGEMENT

The previous two sections of the report should tell the story in general chronological terms about who the client is and how the client arrived at this point in time. Based upon what has been reported before, this section answers the referral question. First, the primary risk factors are identified in a summary paragraph or two. These risk factors should include a recapitulation of those risk factors identified as relevant by the risk appraisal instruments employed. Also included would be risk factors related to the violence outcome of interest that may not be included within the risk appraisal instrument employed. Following this, the actuarial risk estimates are presented along with the instruments from which they were derived. Given the stated risk factors and risk estimate, the release plan is reviewed. We note that release plans may not always be relevant if release is not a possible outcome from the proceedings, but where there is a potential release from an institution, details of the release plans should be clearly delineated. Finally, recommendations for managing risk are presented.

Risk Factors

Recall that in this section you want to recapitulate the primary risk factors of the case, which include those identified by the risk appraisal instrument as well as other relevant risk factors. As an example, consider a situation in which the VRAG was used to estimate actuarial risk with an offender. Below is a sample paragraph that would accomplish this clear identification of risk factors employed by the VRAG. Please note that the *italicized* information in parentheses would not be included in a report but is for instructional purposes here.

> Risk factors identified with Mr. Client include an early onset of inter-personal problems identified by maladjustment in school (*elementary school maladjustment*) and antisocial and criminal behavior in adolescence (*results from the CATS that replaces the PCL-R*). Also, his young age at the time of the offense (*age at index offense*), unmarried status (*marital status*), failure on prior conditional release (*as stated*), and history of prior criminal behavior (*criminal history score for nonviolent offenses*) also present as risk factors. Mr. Client has been diagnosed with antisocial personality disorder (*DSM diagnosis of any personality disorder*) which is also associated with risk for future violence.

A second paragraph could then follow up by identifying those risk factors deemed salient to the case but not necessarily identified by the risk appraisal instrument. Continuing with an example of the OMD consider the following paragraph.

> File information indicated and Mr. Client confirmed that he had two physical altercations with other inmates over the past year. He has also expressed anger verbally toward staff members and has destroyed property when angry while institutionalized. When last in the community he had a history of assaultive behavior resulting in two convictions for battery.

Finally, in the interest of objectivity, thoroughness, and fairness, you should identify important risk factors that may be absent. This is consistent with what some authors refer to as "protective factors" (Rogers, 2000). It has been our experience to date that most protective factors that researchers refer to are ultimately nothing more than the absence of risk factors. For example, some may consider job skills or employment on release a protective factor; however, employment problems have long since been a risk factor so we would consider this an absence of a risk factor.

Actuarial Estimates of Risk

Based upon our discussions in Chapter 4 on the perception and communication of risk information, we are of the opinion that estimates of risk likelihood should be anchored to a numerical probability statement whenever possible. Recall the list of practices that we outlined as the minimum for good risk communication.

1. Name and describe the instrument you are using to estimate risk.

2. Identify that the type of offender from which the predictive norms were derived is consistent for the most part with the individual you are assessing.

3. Describe the outcome of interest. That is, what are you specifically predicting, general recidivism, violent recidivism, or sexual recidivism?

4. Provide the score and the associated estimate of risk for the outcome of interest.

5. Provide the base rate or *average* rate of offending for the outcome of interest. This is important for the decision maker to understand the relative risk the individual represents when compared with the many individuals the decision maker considers. Securing local base rates would be an asset in this regard.

6. Identify any limitations that the instrument may have for the specific case. For example, if an individual is serving a sentence for killing two people and has had no previous convictions for violence and has been well behaved in prison or the institution where he or she was committed, there is a strong likelihood that his or her estimate of risk will be quite low. It will be very important to point out, for example, that instruments like the VRAG or the SORAG were not designed to predict homicide specifically. What they do predict is general violent behavior including robberies, minor and major assaults, and so on. From experience, the primary question in the mind of the decision maker is not whether a murderer will push somebody or rob a corner store (this is likely of secondary interest) but will he or she kill another person if released. The VRAG and the SORAG (or any other instrument we are aware of) will not provide those estimates.

We would also note that some instruments come with the authors' own recommendations for communicating risk. For example, Harris et al. (2007) suggested the following as an approach to communicating the results of the Static-99.

> The recidivism estimates provided by the Static-99 are group estimates based upon reconvictions and were derived from groups of individuals with these characteristics. As such, these estimates do not directly correspond to the recidivism risk of an individual offender. The offender's risk may be higher or lower than the probabilities estimated in the Static-99 depending on other risk factors not measured by this instrument. This instrument should not be used with Young Offenders (those less than 18 years of age) or women.
> Mr. X scored an XX on this risk assessment instrument. Individuals with these characteristics, on average, sexually reoffend at XX% over five years and at XX% over ten years. The rate for any violent recidivism

(including sexual) for individuals with these characteristics is, on average, XX% over five years and XX% over ten years. Based upon the Static-99 score, this places Mr. X in the Low, [score of 0 or 1] (between the 1st and the 23rd percentile); Moderate-Low, [score of 2 or 3] (between the 24th and the 61st percentile); Moderate-High, [score of 4 or 5] (between the 62nd and the 88th percentile); High, [score of 6 plus] (in the top 12%) risk category relative to other adult male sex offenders. (p. 71).

Likewise, Quinsey et al. (2006) also suggested a possible communication strategy (pp. 353–358) for the results of the VRAG and the SORAG. You will notice that these strategies do not include all of the recommendations that we have made above; however, it is up to you as the clinician to decide on the most effective and transparent manner in which to communicate risk, as ultimately you may have to defend your conclusions in legal proceedings.

Release Plans

When a decision is being made to release to the community, the client's release plans become very important. By this time you have identified the risk factors and the associated level of risk that they represent. This is also the case when considering a reduction in security. Taking into consideration where the client could be going and the level of intervention and supervision in that environment deserves important consideration. In this section the task is to identify the proposed destination, whether that is in the community or in a facility with a reduced level of security, and answer the question, Where is the client going to in light of his or her history and pattern of offending? At a minimum you should consider the possible destabilizers, stressors, and social and professional supports as they may interact with the individual's personal vulnerabilities, specifically as they are represented by risk factors.

Recommendations for Managing Risk

Writing a strong Risk Management section is important because it is this section wherein you consider and balance all of the information that has gone before and present it in such a way as to make the information of use to the decision maker. In this section you consider in order the salient risk factors, what if anything has been done so far to address those risk factors, what if anything remains to be accomplished (e.g., intervention, programs), where that intervention can effectively take place (e.g., in their current setting, at a lower security, or in the community), how will the client's current release plan facilitate the needed intervention, what supervision strategies would be most effective, and what level of tolerance if any should there be for noncompliance.

When considering risk factors, you may wish to group together those that are related. For example, employment, education, and financial issues are often related, so these may be treated together as they relate to the client's stability within the community. Similarly, drug and alcohol abuse though sometimes identified separately are generally related. Mental health issues such as stress, emotional functioning, and mood disturbances are different risk factors but are sufficiently related that they could be addressed within risk management strategies together. The integration of related risk factors is intended to balance comprehensiveness with ease of reading for the consumer of the report.

When considering the risk factors, identify what intervention has occurred thus far to address those issues. As an example, when considering the individual's mental health functioning, document what treatment he or she may have received or is currently receiving. This would include medication as well as any structured psychosocial rehabilitation. Where information is available, report the findings of the intervention in terms of compliance, participation, insight, changes in behavior, and how specific the intervention was in addressing that risk factor. Continuing with the same example of mental health issues, you will need to identify what remains to be addressed (new intervention issues) and what needs to be reinforced (maintenance) with respect to managing the mental health concerns. Also important is some comment on where this intervention could be addressed. If a client has addressed the central issues of treating and managing a mood disorder but would benefit from additional psychosocial rehabilitation to maintain the gains made in treatment, it would be helpful to indicate if this maintenance could be accomplished at the lower security or release destination that has been proposed. The central risk issue is not whether every risk factor has been completely addressed, but whether the intervention provided sufficient treatment to manage the client's risk in the destination identified in the decision-making process. This is to avoid the tendency for risk-averse decision makers to insist that the client be "all better" before he or she is released.

In addition your conclusions need to identify supervision strategies and risk situations or circumstances that warrant special attention and intervention should they arise. Supervision strategies are guided by the general principle that the higher the risk, the more intense the supervision and the less tolerance for violations of supervision undertakings. Also identifying key circumstances or symptoms that warrant immediate intervention such as the deterioration in mental illness symptoms for offenders with mental illness, the close proximity of sex offenders to their victim pool, or the beginnings of an intimate relationship for a spouse abuser may all be risk factors that those supervising these very different offenders may need to know about that would warrant intervention or at the least closer supervision.

When working with OMDs, functional impairments, such as not paying fines, may contribute, indirectly, to the relationship between mental illness and failure (Skeem & Eno Louden, 2006). This finding is consistent with the literature reviewed thus far and highlights the necessity of practical and reasonable suggestions for risk management of OMDs. One applicable suggestion includes supervision strategies to decrease anxiety, perceived threat, and negative affect.

Skeem et al. (2004) also pointed out an important consideration for risk management strategies among OMDs by showing that not all high-risk patients are the same. Specifically, they identified three distinct groups; the first group was depressed, abused drugs heavily, had extensive histories of arrest, and had multiple psychopathic characteristics. The second group was dysphoric, dependent on alcohol or drugs, and sensitive to personal problems with relatively good histories of adjustment. The third group had delusional experiences, less drug and alcohol involvement, experienced command hallucinations, and had histories of intensive treatment. Thus, for the first group treatment targets would include substance abuse and negative affect. Also, this group would benefit from a focus on psychopathic traits. The second group will benefit from substance abuse treatment, and from coping, negative affect, and self-regulation skills. The third group will benefit from treating the positive symptoms of psychosis.

With offender samples, the occurrence of comorbidity is very common. In examining the prevalence of comorbidity among offenders, Blackburn, Logan, Donnelly, and Renwick (2003) found that OMDs diagnosed with Axis I illness also had a personality disorder. This was true regardless of the mode of assessment (interview schedule vs. self-report). Similarly, the converse was also true. Those with a personality disorder reported one or more Axis I disorders in the past, with 50% having an active Axis I disorder. When examining psychopathy, there was no evidence that psychopathy was associated with higher level of Axis I disorders. In summary there is no single, unique pattern for OMDs. Recommendation for managing risk will account for individual differences among OMDs.

TESTIFYING IN LEGAL PROCEEDINGS

Owing to the typical goal and purpose of violence risk assessments, it is likely that clinicians providing this service will, at some point in time, be called to testify in legal proceedings (e.g., court, parole hearing). There are many excellent references for preparing to testify in court, references that are applicable to other legal proceedings as well (cf. Brodsky 1991, 1999, 2004;

Melton et al., 2007). Readers are encouraged to peruse these resources well in advance of preparation for court. When time is of the essence, however, and you have limited time to prepare your testimony, we provide here recommendations for improving the probability of a successful experience.

Preparing to Testify

Preparing to testify in court is much simpler if you have had an occasion to consult with the attorney calling for your testimony. A pretrial conference is "highly recommended" (p. 588) because it provides invaluable information regarding the strategy of direct examination (*direct examination* is questioning by the attorney who called the expert to court; Melton et al., 2007). In addition to outlining the case an attorney will identify strategies that allow the psychologist to help the case (Hess, 2006). This exchange not only provides the psychologist with a preview of the line of questioning to expect, but also affords the astute psychologist an opportunity to identify the motives of the attorney (truth seeking or seeking a hired gun), as well as his or her conceptualization of the case and the attorney's ability to create a favorable first impression, an important consideration given that the effectiveness of an expert's testimony is tied to the skills and abilities of the attorney examining him or her (Hess, 2006). Finally, the pretrial conference provides an opportunity for the expert and the attorney to agree on the "ultimate-issue" issue. That is, you should make the attorney aware of your position with regard to ultimate-issue testimony (*ultimate issue* refers to mental health professionals providing opinions or conclusions that address the ultimate legal issue; readers are referred to Melton et al., 2007, for a detailed discussion of this subject).

Even if you participated in a pretrial conference, your preparation is not yet finished. Prior to providing testimony you should carefully review all relevant assessment materials to include records obtained from third-party sources, interview and collateral informant notes, results of psychological testing, and of course the written report(s) if reports were developed. Although it can be beneficial for purposes of impression management for the expert to admit not knowing some information (e.g., not having read a research paper published by another expert, not being familiar with an obscure psychological theory), this does not extend to the nature of the experts' risk assessment, sources of conclusions, and opinions. The expert should be readily able to respond to questions directly tied to one's evaluation and nothing can better prepare the expert for presenting as an expert to the fact finder (e.g., judge, jury, parole board) than intensive pretrial review of the case record.

When called to testify, you will be queried, either formally, such as in a court of law, or more informally, such as in a parole hearing, as to your knowledge and expertise to perform the risk assessment and provide conclusions and opinions based on that evaluation. This process is referred to as *voir dire* and simply refers to the process of qualifying you as an expert. This process can be greatly enhanced by providing the attorney who called you to testify with a list of your credentials and prepared questions during the pretrial conference. In general, voir dire will (1) review your formal education including dates, degrees obtained, and titles of academic research projects if applicable; (2) provide the fact finder a summary of your practical experiences to include postdoctoral fellowships, internships, practica completed, as well as professional positions to date; (3) professional certifications and licensures obtained; (4) professional memberships (e.g., American Psychological Association, American Psychology – Law Society, Canadian Psychological Association); (5) research record including research awards (i.e., grants), books written, and professional publications and presentations; and (6) previous experience as an expert witness (Melton et al., 2007).

Following voir dire you will undergo direct examination followed by cross-examination. Much has been written about the tactics used by skilled attorneys during cross-examination; however, once you have become familiar with these tactics and developed strategies for dealing with them when they occur, you can relax and begin to enjoy your role as informant to the fact finder (Melton et al., 2007). For a review of these tactics and effective strategies for countering them, see the previously recommended sources of Brodsky (1991, 1999, 2004) and Melton et al. (2007).

Based on our experience, a few additional words of caution are warranted. First, you would be naive to enter the legal arena without considering issues of impression management. To be effective in legal settings (trials and hearings, depositions, etc.), you simply must dress appropriately. More broadly, you need to appreciate and follow courtroom protocol, including how to address the jury, judge, or parole board. Learn what is known about what it takes to communicate effectively, and familiarize yourself with the general social psychology literature on credibility (cf. Melton et al., 2007). For example, you should train yourself to speak to the fact finder following questioning by the attorney. A lack of attention to simple etiquette and an inability to manage others' impressions of you as an expert will result in less effective testimony.

Maintaining Your Composure

A discussion of providing expert testimony would not be complete without a discussion of composure. Simply stated, it is your responsibility to maintain your composure when testifying, including during cross-examination, which can become quite adversarial. If you lose your composure, you will lose credibility with the fact finder and will be much less effective. We have found it much easier to maintain composure when we are relieved of the internal pressure of defending our findings and opinions. We assume it is not our job during direct or cross-examination to defend our findings, conclusions, or opinions. Rather, it is our role to clarify any misunderstandings regarding our findings, conclusions, and opinions. That includes occasions when attorneys present "new information" during cross-examination. Rather than clinging to our reported conclusions, we should consider any new data in light of preexisting data and revise our conclusions and opinions accordingly. Granted, new data rarely results in revised conclusions or opinions, but this mind-set of being open to new information and simply directing your responses in a manner to inform and educate the fact finder relieves much of the pressure many experts wrongly place on themselves to defend their findings.

We have also found it beneficial to recognize that cross-examination is not personal. The attorney who challenges you is simply doing his or her job to represent his or her position. This will often mean the attorney must "attack" an expert's findings and opinions, but note that skilled attorneys will rarely attack an expert directly. In our experience, when an attorney directs his or her attacks to the expert, it means the attorney has no basis for attacking the merits of the expert's findings, conclusions, and opinions. If you weather such an attack, which most often simply requires maintaining your composure, then you can rest assured that the attorney has little else to follow up with.

The criminal justice system and its components (courts, parole hearings, and other legal arenas in which you may find yourself providing testimony after conducting a violence risk assessment) are adversarial by design. If you can appreciate this system and recognize the benefits of it, and the respective roles of those asking you questions, it will be much simpler to maintain a positive and productive mind-set (and thereby your composure), as you will not be undone by tactics designed to divert your attention away from the task at hand.

APPENDIX

■   ■   ■

SAMPLE VIOLENCE RISK ASSESSMENT

[This report sample is based on an assessment of an incarcerated offender who will soon be considered for a conditional release by a parole board. The risk assessment is a part of the decision-making process when considering the release of an individual who has a history of violent offending.]

Name:	John D. Client
Date of Birth:	September 1, 1969
Institution:	Fictitious Correctional Facility
Date Sentence Commenced:	October 1, 2006
Date of Report:	September 4, 2009

ASSESSMENT CONTEXT

Referral

Mr. Client is a 40-year-old federally sentenced offender serving a sentence of 4 years, 6 months for the offenses of robbery and failure to appear. Mr. Client has had prior convictions for violent behavior. Mr. Client is soon to be considered for parole, and the parole board will consider a possible supervised release to the community. In keeping with parole board policy, due to his violent behavior, a violence risk assessment has been requested by his parole officer, Mr. Smith, of Fictitious Correctional Facility. The purpose of this assessment is to identify risk factors for general and violent offending, provide an estimate of the likelihood for recidivism, and identify strategies for managing that risk.

Evaluation Process

This assessment is based upon a 2-hour interview with Mr. Client in the Psychology Department at Fictitious Correctional Facility on September 1, 2009. Additionally, Mr. Client completed a number of psychometric tests on August 26, 2009, which are detailed below. The case management, discipline, psychology, and medical files were made available to me, and documents of particular relevance are detailed below. The risk appraisal instruments employed in this evaluation include the Level of Service Inventory—Revised (Andrews & Bonta, 1995) and the Risk Management Indicators of the Two-Tiered Violence Risk Estimates (Mills & Kroner, 2005).

Psychometric Testing

    Wechsler Fundamentals Academic Skills
    Personality Assessment Inventory (Morey, 2007)
    Measures of Antisocial Attitudes and Associates (Mills, Kroner, & Forth, 2002)
    Criminal Attributions Inventory (Kroner & Mills, 2002)

File Information

Release Planning Report	I. Smith	July 3, 2009
Community Assessment	F. Banks	May 24, 2009
Correctional Progress Report	G. Thomas	November 10, 2008
Substance Abuse Treatment Evaluation	D. Jones	May 2, 2008
Discipline Report	K. McIntyre	June 23, 2007
Correctional Plan	C. Bell	February 14, 2007
Intake Evaluation	B. Miles	December 12, 2006
Judge's Reason for Sentencing		
Police Reports		

Consent

Prior to the commencement of taking the psychometric tests, Mr. Client had an opportunity to read and voluntarily sign a consent form outlining the purpose, nature, and process of the assessment; the party for whom the assessment was being completed; the limits of confidentiality; my mandatory reporting requirements; and his right to withdraw at any time. I reviewed with Mr. Client the contents of the form, at which time he evidenced understanding of the issues and indicated his consent by signing the form. I determined from our discussion at that time that Mr. Client understood clearly the process and implications and was competent to give informed consent.

Interview Impressions

Mr. Client's responses to questions were appropriately as descriptive and brief as the question required. Mr. Client presented himself in an open fashion and provided information about himself that was both positive and negative. He did not attempt to evade answering questions and was direct in his responses. There were indications of impression management from his responses to questions regarding prior violent behavior. His version of his criminal record tended to differ from the official versions, and he either denied the offense or portrayed himself as much less culpable than the court findings would indicate. His reporting of the events surrounding the current crime for which he is sentenced is consistent with official documents. There were no contradictions in self-report. His accompanying affect was appropriate to the content of the interview. There were no deficits in self-care. There were no overt symptoms of psychological or psychiatric disorders. His memory appeared intact, and he showed no difficulty in placing events within chronological order and remembered relevant dates and times. Mr. Client was well oriented to person, time, and place, and did not express any disturbed thoughts, delusional thinking, or suicidal/homicidal ideation.

PSYCHOSOCIAL BACKGROUND

Family of Origin, Childhood, and Adolescence

Mr. Client was born in Montreal, Quebec, and raised in an intact biological family. He quickly identified himself as the "black sheep" of the family. He reported that his parents remained married until his father's death 2 years ago. His three siblings are all independent and living with families of their own. He indicated that he maintains regular contact with his mother and his younger sister through letters and the occasional phone call. His said that his older brother and sister have little to do with him as they view him as an "embarrassment" to the family.

Mr. Client had predominantly fond memories of his childhood. He said that in hindsight he recognized how hard his parents worked to provide for the family. He said that they did not have a lot of material possessions in the initial years but they were never without food or clothing. Mr. Client recalled that he began exhibiting behavioral problems as he approached his teenage years.

Mr. Client recalled that both his parents worked to provide financially for the family after emigrating from the United Kingdom. Because of the economic challenges the family faced they initially resided in a low-rent district, which he describes as a "bad neighborhood." He recalled that drugs were readily accessible at his school, and physical confrontations among students were frequent. As the family's economic situation improved, his parents eventually moved them to a middle-class neighborhood when he was 14 years of age. He described difficulty adjusting to the move, and he maintained regular contact with his friends from his old neighborhood.

Despite a positive home environment absent of verbal, emotional, physical, or sexual abuse or neglect, he began to have conflict with his parents after he and his friends were caught shoplifting when he was 11 years old. He acknowledged that he seemed to gravitate to the "wrong crowd." By the age of 12 he was sneaking alcohol from his parents' home. He also related that he would defy his parents and sneak out of the home when grounded. Despite the change in neighborhood Mr. Client would return to his friends in his old neighborhood with regularity. By the age of 14 years, Mr. Client was skipping school, regularly smoking cannabis, and running into conflict with the law for shoplifting, possession of narcotics, and misdemeanor offenses.

Education, Employment, and Financial History

Mr. Client said that he terminated his education when he was 16 years old. He reported many periods of truancy prior to quitting school, which he attributed to the time spent with his friends. He recalled being suspended once for fighting and once for bringing alcohol to school. He stated that he was expelled before finishing the 10th grade after throwing a book at a teacher. Mr. Client said that he informed his parents one day that he would not be returning to school, and the parents did not force the issue. Test results from the Wechsler Fundamentals Academic Skills, administered as part of this assessment, placed Mr. Client's reading skills at the grade 8 level, his spelling skills at the grade 5 level, and his arithmetic skills at the grade 6 level.

After leaving school Mr. Client remained in his parent's home for 2 years. He said that his parents insisted that he have a job, so he found part-time work. These jobs rarely lasted for more than a few months at a time before he either quit or was fired. He recalled that during his teenage years he lost two jobs due to being in jail for brief periods of time. As an adult Mr. Client does not recall maintaining a full-time job for a 1-year period. He listed a number of jobs he held for various periods of time, none of which lasted more than 9 months. He supported himself primarily through social assistance which has been augmented by crime (stolen goods, selling marijuana); at times he relied on the support of intimate partners.

Marital/Intimate Relationships

Mr. Client reported that his first sexual experience was at the age of 15 with a same-age female partner. He indicated that he had a number of girlfriends during his teenage years but none of these relationships lasted beyond a few months until he met the woman he would eventually marry. Mr. Client reported that he was always faithful to the women he was involved with, though he did indicate he had a number of casual sexual relationships. He informed me that his sexual relationships have all been consensual with appropriate-age female partners.

There was no file information to indicate that Mr. Client has engaged in inappropriate sexual behavior.

Mr. Client reported that he has been married twice and most recently has been in a common-law relationship for the past 4 years. He was first married when he was 20 years old to a young woman who was 17 years old at the time. He said that they were married after she became pregnant with their child. The marriage lasted about 3 years and produced two children, a boy now 20 years old and a girl now 18 years old. Mr. Client said that the relationship ended because of his alcohol abuse. In hindsight he feels his wife grew tired of waiting for him to "grow up," and she ended the relationship when she discovered he had been unfaithful. His second marriage occurred when he was 25 years old and lasted less than a year. Again he cited his alcohol abuse for the reason the relationship ended. He reported that he was able to keep his drinking under control for periods of time but eventually he would return to drinking every day, and this strained his relationships. Mr. Client said that he has had a number of common-law relationships in the intervening years, none lasting more than 3 years. He has two more children, a boy of 12 and a girl of 8, each with a different woman. He reported that his most stable relationship has been the relationship he currently has with a woman who is 2 years his junior. She has two children from a previous relationship, two girls, one 12 and the other 15.

Mr. Client reported that his relationships started out amicable but often deteriorated into arguments and conflict when his alcohol consumption increased or when financial problems arose. He was quite clear that these arguments never became physical as he would leave the home before "things got out of hand."

Substance Use/Abuse

Mr. Client said he began drinking when he was 11 years old when some of his friends would steal alcohol from home. He would drink mostly when with his friends, but as he grew older he began to drink on his own. He recalled that during his teenage years he spent most weekends at a "party" where he would consume alcohol to intoxication. It was not until he was in his 20s that he increased his alcohol consumption to weekdays and eventually every day. He reported daily alcohol use except when it was interrupted by incarceration. Mr. Client reported that he began to smoke marijuana when he was 14 years old. He described his teenage use of marijuana as "recreational" at parties. He said that he has smoked marijuana at least once a week for most of his adult life. He recalled that he would support this drug use by selling marijuana to friends on a "small scale." He denied ever selling large quantities of drugs.

Mr. Client reported that he stopped his alcohol use about 4 years ago when he met his current partner. According to Mr. Client, his partner is a former alcoholic who made it clear that she would have nothing to do with alcohol and nothing to do with him if he drank. He said that he has remained sober for the past 4 years, though he has smoked marijuana with friends when "it was available," though never around his partner.

Mr. Client said he first used cocaine about 3 months prior to his arrest on the charges for which he is currently sentenced. He said his partner was away from home visiting her parents when he spent some time with a friend, and they smoked marijuana. Mr. Client related that his friend introduced him to cocaine during this time, and his use of the drug quickly escalated to almost daily over the next month. Within the following 2 months Mr. Client said that his life revolved around cocaine use. Mr. Client reported that he and his coaccused had been using cocaine very heavily for 3 days when they ran out of both money and drugs. He recalled that on the day of the offense they robbed a jewelry store quite spontaneously. Mr. Client also reported that prior to the offense he had been spending hundreds of dollars each day and selling marijuana to fund his cocaine use.

Attitudes, Associates, and Attributions

Mr. Client said that he has had criminal associates through most of his life. At a superficial level he understands they have not been helpful, but he fails to grasp the influence his associates have had on him over the years. Mr. Client did not express any directly overt antisocial attitudes, though there were instances when he employed rationalizations and to a lesser extent justifications to explain why he continued to use alcohol and drugs and why he continued to remain involved in the criminal subculture. Mr. Client's responses to the Measures of Criminal Attitudes and Associates scale were quite consistent with other offenders. His attitudes of entitlement, attitudes toward violence and criminal others, and expressions of antisocial intent all fell within the normative range when compared with other federally incarcerated offenders. He identified that two of the people he spends the most time with have been involved in criminal activities. Mr. Client also completed the Criminal Attributions Inventory, and his responses indicated that he tends to blame substance abuse and psychopathology for criminal behavior, and less so personal attributes, victims, and society. He also endorsed items that indicate crime is caused by random events or chance. Taken together with the interview content, Mr. Client left the impression that he tended to rationalize or excuse crime as somewhat out of his control.

With respect to his sentence, Mr. Client feels that it was relatively fair though "a little harsh" and does not appear to have a negative view of the criminal justice system. He accepts responsibility for his offense, with the aforementioned tendency to mitigate the behavior.

Leisure

Mr. Client said that prior to his 3 months of cocaine use he spent his free time with his partner and her two children. He would occasionally meet with friends at a local mall as he was trying to stay away from bars and roadhouses. He did report that prior to his current relationship he tended to spend more time with friends, mostly other criminals or alcoholics, in generally idle and nonproductive activities. He has no recreational or leisure interests. He would visit his mother and younger sister regularly, though he would avoid family gatherings because of the friction between him and his older siblings.

Psychological/Mental Health Functioning

Mr. Client said that he has never been in the care of a mental health professional. He indicated that shortly after his arrival to custody on the current charges he experienced symptoms of depression and was prescribed medication by the institutional physician. He could not recall if a diagnosis was made and there is no record of a diagnosis on his file. Within 6 months he stopped taking the medication as he believed he no longer needed it. He could not recall any periods of time where he experienced significant mood disturbance. He provided no information to suggest the presence of mental illness either past or present. He reported that he experienced passive thoughts of suicide shortly after his arrest, but these ideations did not last once he detoxified following the cocaine binge. There were no other indicators of risk for self-harm evident during our interview.

Results from the Personality Assessment Inventory indicate that Mr. Client approached the test with a tendency to present himself in a favorable light. Other validity indices were within normal limits. There were no significant elevations among the clinical scales, which is consistent with an absence of serious mental illness. Mr. Client's responses suggest a measure of impulsivity and egocentricity. His profile is consistent with someone who has been in conflict with the law. A moderate elevation in the area of verbal aggression is noted and is consistent with someone who would readily display anger and not back down from confrontation. Mr. Client reports that drugs have posed a significant problem in his life. Overall Mr. Client's responses are quite consistent with his presentation during the interview and information gleaned from file information.

HISTORY OF VIOLENCE AND CRIMINAL BEHAVIOR

Offense History

Juvenile Record: Theft (March 4, 1984), Possession of Stolen Property (June 15, 1984), Mischief (September 17, 1984), Possession of Narcotics (January 16, 1985).

Adult Convictions: Driving with More Than 80mg (September 3, 1989), Fail to Appear (x2) (September 17, 1989), Assault Causing Bodily Harm (March 17, 1990), Theft of Auto, Dangerous Driving (August 10, 1995), Theft Over, Public Mischief (October 7, 1998), Theft Over, Fail to Comply (January 3, 2000), Uttering Threats (x4), Assault with Weapon, Assault, Fail to Attend, Fail to Comply (May 9, 2001), Robbery, Fail to Appear (October 1, 2006).

Mr. Client said that the Assault Causing Bodily Harm in 1990 was associated with a fight he had with a patron in his role as a pub bouncer. He said the bar patron hit him when he refused him entry for not meeting the dress code. Mr. Client said that he pursued the patron outside of the establishment and beat him up.

With respect to the threats in 2001, Mr. Client admitted that he threatened to beat someone up who had been saying malicious things about him within the community. However, police reports indicate a pattern of violent threats against various individuals in the community with whom Mr. Client had taken issue, and that the threats were of death.

Mr. Client said that the assaults in 2001 were related to the same period of time and issues. He said that the assault with a weapon never happened. He stated quite emphatically that he was at a party when he became embroiled in a heated argument with another person. Both men were intoxicated at the time. Mr. Client said that the he confronted the other man as the man was doing extensive damage to his car with a cast iron frying pan. He reported that he gained the upper hand in the ensuing fight and he took the pan from the other man. Coincidentally, the police arrived at the moment he took that pan, and he was charged with assault with a weapon. Police reports indicated that the other man was seriously hurt and sustained among other injuries blunt force bruising to the abdomen and arms. In the other instance of assault, Mr. Client said that while drinking at a bar an acquaintance kicked him in the chest and then fell backward to the floor. He was again charged but said that he did not assault the other man. Police reports indicated that it was Mr. Client who did the kicking and subsequently threw a beer bottle at the victim.

Current Offense

Mr. Client recounted the events surrounding the current offense and readily accepts responsibility for his actions. He related that he and his coaccused had been on a cocaine binge and when they ran out of both money and drugs impulsively decided to rob a jewelry store. Mr. Client blames his heavily intoxicated state for the offense. He said he cannot remember all of the details but does recall that he entered the store and pretended to be armed. He forced the store clerks into the back room, where the safe happened to be open.

He and his coaccused filled two plastic bags with jewelry and fled the premises. There appears to be some contradiction in official reports as to the amount stolen. An occurrence report dated March 21, 2006, indicated that $15,000 worth of jewelry was taken from the store safe.

Institutional Behavior

Mr. Client has incurred one institutional offense to date. He said that he bought a television from another offender who was being released. Correctional officers searching his cell charged him with having an unauthorized item in his cell as the television was not listed among his belongings. Mr. Client admitted candidly to his actions and said that the television he purchased was better than the one he had at the time. He is currently undertaking high school studies through the institutional school, and while his motivation, attendance, and interpersonal relationships have been very good his progress has been slow.

Mr. Client also attended the Offender Substance Abuse Program. This is a 12-week cognitive-behavioral-based group intervention that requires daily attendance for approximately 2 hours each session. The program is quite structured and includes motivational interviewing and preparation, skill acquisition, problem solving, release planning, and relapse prevention. The program report indicated that Mr. Client was a good participant who was usually prompt with homework assignments. He appeared to grasp the main elements though he had some difficulty developing his relapse prevention plan.

Prior Release Behavior

Mr. Client has had multiple release opportunities during periods of probation and bail. He has also failed to meet his conditions of release on a number of occasions, and this has resulted in additional criminal convictions.

RISK ASSESSMENT AND RISK MANAGEMENT

Risk Factors

Mr. Client reported a serious and chronic alcohol abuse problem, though he reportedly (unconfirmed) remained sober for a significant period of time prior to the current offense.

Despite his abstinence from alcohol he continued to use marijuana on occasion. It was his continued association with drug
users that appears to have led to a brief but intense cocaine
addiction that is directly related to his current offense.

Mr. Client's interpersonal relationships have tended to be
brief and by his own admission tumultuous. He attributed
these difficulties to his chronic abuse of alcohol over the
years. He has a long history of associating with other criminals and drug users.

In addition, Mr. Client acts impulsively when confronted by
problems. His repertoire of responses includes threats and
assault, suggesting quite strongly the presence of attitudes that view violence or the threat of violence acceptable. The early onset of antisocial and criminal activity,
which persisted throughout adolescence and into adulthood,
reflects an entrenched antisocial behavior pattern. Adolescent fights and later adult charges for assault also speak
to the issue of a prolonged behavior pattern that includes
violence.

A poor academic background, conflicts in school, later difficulty in maintaining self-supporting employment, and unproductive leisure activities are all risk factors associated
with a criminal lifestyle and the perseverance of this behavior pattern over time.

Actuarial Estimates of Risk

Mr. Client's responses were also scored according to the
Level of Service Inventory—Revised (LSI-R). This is a risk
appraisal instrument designed to provide indicators of criminal risk, in order to estimate risk and determine supervision
levels. Mr. Client's score was 36 on this instrument. As a
group, 57.3% of offenders with a similar score will reoffend
within approximately 2 years. The average rate of recidivism
for the group on which the LSI-R was developed was approximately 40.8%. However, this group of offenders on which these
original estimates are based were serving sentences of less
than 2 years. Other research has shown that the same score
with federal offenders serving greater than 2 years was associated with a 68% likelihood to reoffend over a 3-year period,
with the average rate of reoffending for the comparison group
being 49% (see Mills, Jones, & Kroner, 2005).

Mr. Client's personal and criminal history was scored on the Two-Tiered Violence Risk Estimate (TTV). The TTV was developed to assist in determining the level of risk for violence in male offenders. Mr. Client's score was 11 on this instrument. As a group, other offenders with a similar score will reoffend violently (assault, robbery, assault with a weapon, etc.) at a rate between 31 and 46% over a 3-year period of time. The average rate of offending for the comparison group of offenders was 29% over a 3-year period.

In general, the actuarial measures place Mr. Client's likelihood to reoffend at a rate above that of the average offender for both general and violent recidivism.

Release Plans

At the present time, Mr. Client plans to return to his partner and her home as she remains his primary community support. He said that he will likely attend Alcoholics Anonymous when released, as he has been to a number of meetings while incarcerated. He reports that his younger sister has promised she will try to find him a job in the loading docks of the company for whom she currently works.

Recommendations for Managing Risk

Mr. Client is encouraged to continue with his high school studies while incarcerated. Upon release there would be a definite long-term personal benefit if he could obtain his high school diploma or equivalency. His work history has been inconsistent and he has been unable to secure and maintain self-supporting employment. Prior to his current offense he was supported primarily by his partner as he was only able to secure part-time employment stocking shelves at a local supermarket. His long-term success will require him to develop employment skills sufficient to maintain an unskilled or manual labor job.

Mr. Client has a history of breaches of trust and failure to comply with conditions of release. Therefore, any release to the community should be accompanied by intensive supervision with a zero tolerance for violations of any conditions of release. Indications of noncompliance with supervision (failing to report on time, not being forthcoming with information to his parole supervisor) or conditions of release should be considered an indication of a closer proximity to reoffending.

According to Mr. Client, alcohol and drug abuse has been a contributing factor to his criminal offending. He has completed the Offender Substance Abuse Program while incarcerated, and overall the program report was positive. Nonetheless, his relapse prevention planning was considered to require additional work and was considered his weakest area in terms of program goal attainment. It is important that Mr. Client receive ongoing support to maintain his sobriety and drug abstinence while in the community. A community-based program, inpatient or halfway house preferably, would assist Mr. Client in making the adjustment to the community with respect to his addictions and also provide the addition of extra supervision. It would be prudent to include a condition to abstain from alcohol and nonprescribed medication as part of Mr. Client's release. Evidence that Mr. Client has returned to using alcohol or cocaine should be considered an indication of a closer proximity for reoffending.

Antisocial and criminal associations have contributed significantly to Mr. Client's criminal behavior by reinforcing criminal values behavior. If available, programing or therapy that would address antisocial attitudes and associates would be an asset. It would also be prudent to include as a condition of release a requirement for Mr. Client to refrain from associating with anyone known to have a criminal record or to be engaging in criminal behavior.

I trust this assessment will assist you in your evaluation. If there are further clarifications or specific questions I can address on the basis of my examination of Mr. Client, please contact me at your convenience.

Respectfully,

_____   _____
Clinician name and credentials   Date

REFERENCES

Abel, G. G., Gore, D. K., Holland, C. L., Camp, N., Becker, J. V., & Rather, J. (1989). The measurement of the cognitive distortions in child molesters. *Annals of Sex Research, 2,* 135–153.

Addison v. Texas, 441 U.S. 418 (1979).

Aegisdottir, S., White, M. J., Spengler, P. M., Maugherman, A. S., Anderson, L. A., Nichols, C. N., et al. (2006). The Meta-Analysis of Clinical Judgment Project: Fifty-six years of accumulated research on clinical versus statistical prediction. *Counseling Psychologist, 34,* 341–382.

Aldridge, M. L., & Browne, K. D. (2003). Perpetrators of spousal homicide: A review. *Trauma, Violence, and Abuse, 4,* 265–276.

Allan, M., Grace, R. C., Rutherford, B., & Hudson, S. M. (2007). Psychometric assessment of dynamic risk factors for child molesters. *Sex Abuse, 19,* 347–367.

American Psychiatric Association. (1994). *Diagnostic and statistical manual of mental disorders* (4th ed.). Washington, DC: Author.

American Psychiatric Association. (2000). *Diagnostic and statistical manual of mental disorders* (4th ed., text rev.). Washington, DC: Author.

Andrews, D. A. (1982). *The Level of Supervision Inventory (LSI): The first follow-up.* Toronto: Ministry of Correctional Services of Ontario.

Andrews, D. A., & Bonta, J. (1995). *The Level of Service Inventory—Revised (Manual).* Toronto: Multi-Health Systems.

Andrews, D. A., & Bonta, J. (1998). *The psychology of criminal conduct* (2nd ed.). Cincinnati: Anderson.

Andrews, D. A., & Bonta, J. (2010). *The psychology of criminal conduct* (5th ed.). New Providence, NJ: LexisNexis Group.

Andrews, D. A., Bonta, J., & Wormith, J. S. (1995). *Level of Service Inventory—Ontario Revision (LSI-OR): Interview and scoring guide.* Toronto: Ontario Ministry of the Solicitor General and Correctional Services.

Andrews, D. A., Bonta, J., & Wormith, J. S. (2004). *Manual for the Level of Service/Case Management Inventory (LS/CMI).* Toronto: Multi-Health Systems.

Andrews, D. A., Bonta, J., & Wormith, J. S. (2006). The recent past and near future of risk and/or need assessment. *Crime and Delinquency, 52,* 7–27.

Andrews, D. A., & Dowden, C. (2005). Managing correctional treatment for reduced recidivism: A meta-analytic review of program integrity. *Legal and Criminological Psychology, 10,* 173–187.

Andrews, D. A., & Robinson, D. (1984). *The Level of Supervision Inventory: Second report.* Toronto: Ministry of Correctional Services of Ontario.

Andrews, D. A., Zinger, I., Hoge, R. D., Bonta, J., Gendreau, P., & Cullen, F. T. (1990). Does correctional treatment work?: A clinically relevant and psychologically informed meta-analysis. *Criminology, 28,* 369–404.

Aos, S., Phipps, P., Barnoski, R., & Lieb, R. (2001). *The comparative costs and benefits of programs to reduce crime* (Version 4.0). Olympia, WA: Washington State Institute for Public Policy.

Appelbaum, P. S., Robbins, P. C., & Monahan, J. (2000). Violence and delusions: Data from the MacArthur Violence Risk Assessment Study. *American Journal of Psychiatry, 157,* 566–572.

Appelbaum, P. S., & Grisso, T. (1988). Assessing patients' capacities to consent to treatment. *New England Journal of Medicine, 319,* 1635–1638.

Arboleda-Flórez, J. (1998). Mental illness and violence: An epidemiological appraisal of the evidence. *Canadian Journal of Psychiatry, 43,* 989–996.

Arseneault, L., Moffitt, T. E., Caspi, A., Taylor, P. J., & Silva, P. A. (2000). Mental disorders and violence in a total birth cohort: Results from the Dunedin Study. *Archives of General Psychiatry, 57,* 979–986.

Austin, J. (2006). How much risk can we take?: The misuse of risk assessment in corrections. *Federal Probation, 70,* 58–63.

Banks, S., Clark-Robbins, P., Silver, E., Vesselinov, R., Steadman, H. J., Monahan, J., et al. (2004). A multiple-models approach to violence risk assessment among people with mental disorder. *Criminal Justice and Behavior, 31,* 324–340.

Barbaree, H. E., & Marshall, W. L. (Eds.). (2008). *The juvenile sex offender* (2nd ed.). New York: Guilford Press.

Barbaree, H. E., Seto, M. C., Langton, C. M., & Peacock, E. J. (2001). Evaluating the predictive accuracy of six risk assessment instruments for adult sex offenders. *Criminal Justice and Behavior, 28,* 490–521.

Bartosh, D. L., Garby, T., Lewis, D., & Gray, S. (2003). Differences in the predictive validity of actuarial risk assessment in relation to sex offender type. *International Journal of Offender Therapy and Comparative Criminology, 47,* 422–438.

Bassuk, E. L., Buckner, J. C., Weinreb, L. F., Browne, A., Bassuk, S. S., Dawson, R., et al. (1997). Homelessness in female-headed families: Childhood and adult risk and protective factors. *American Journal of Public Health, 87,* 241–248.

Beal, C. A., Kroner, D. G., & Weekes, J. R. (2003). Persecutory ideation and depression in mild violence among incarcerated adult males. *International Journal of Offender Therapy and Comparative Criminology, 47,* 159–170.

Beck, A. T., Steer, R. A., & Brown, G. K. (1997). *Beck Depression Inventory—2nd Edition manual.* San Antonio, TX: Psychological Corporation.

Beech, A. R. (1998). A psychometric typology of child abusers. *International Journal of Offender Therapy and Comparative Criminology, 42,* 319–339,

Belfrage, H., Fransson, G., & Strand, S. (2000). Prediction of violence using the HCR-20: A prospective study in two maximum-security correctional institutions. *Journal of Forensic Psychiatry, 11*, 167–175.

Bengtson, S., & Langstrom, N. (2007). Unguided clinical and actuarial assessment of reoffending risk: A direct comparison with sex offenders in Denmark. *Sex Abuse, 19*, 135–153.

Blackburn, R., Donnelly, J. P., Logan, C., & Renwick, S. J. D. (2004). Convergent and discriminative validity of interview and questionnaire measures of personality disorder in mentally disordered offenders: A multitrait-multimethod analysis using confirmatory factor analysis. *Journal of Personality Disorders, 18*, 129–150.

Blackburn, R., Logan, C., Donnelly, J., & Renwick, S. (2003). Personality disorders, psychopathy and other mental disorders: Co-mobidity among patients at English and Scottish high-security hospitals. *Journal of Forensic Psychiatry and Psychology, 14*, 111–137.

Blancette, K., & Brown, S. L. (2006). *The assessment and treatment of women offenders: An integrative perspective.* West Sussex, UK: Wiley.

Boer, D. P., Hart, S. D., Kropp, P. R., & Webster, C. D. (1997). *Manual for the Sexual Violence Risk-20: Professional guidelines for assessing risk of sexual violence.* Vancouver: Mental Health, Law, and Policy Institute, Simon Fraser University.

Bonta, J. (1989, January). Native inmates: Institutional response, risk, and needs. *Canadian Journal of Criminology*, 49–62.

Bonta, J. (2002). Offender risk assessment: Guidelines for selection and use. *Criminal Justice and Behavior, 29*, 355–379.

Bonta, J., Harman, W. G., Hann, R. G., & Cormier, R. B. (1996). The prediction of recidivism among federally sentenced offenders: A re-validation of the SIR scale. *Canadian Journal of Criminology, 38*, 61–79.

Bonta, J., LaPraire, C., & Wallace-Capretta, S. (1997). Risk prediction and re-offending: Aboriginal and non-aboriginal offenders. *Canadian Journal of Criminology, 39*, 127–144.

Bonta, J., Law, M., & Hanson, K. (1998). The prediction of criminal and violent recidivism among mentally disordered offenders: A meta-analysis. *Psychological Bulletin, 123*, 123–142.

Bonta, J., & Motiuk, L. L. (1987). The diversion of incarcerated offenders to correctional halfway houses. *Journal of Research in Crime and Delinquency, 24*, 302–323.

Bonta, J., & Motiuk, L. L. (1990). Classification to correctional halfway houses: A quasi-experimental evaluation. *Criminology, 28*, 497–506.

Borum, R. (1996). Improving the clinical practice of violence risk assessment: Technology, guidelines, and training. *American Psychologist, 51*, 945–956.

Borum, R., & Reddy, M. (2001). Assessing violence risk in Tarasoff situations: A fact-based model of inquiry. *Behavioral Sciences and the Law, 19*, 375–385.

Borum, R., & Verhaagen, D. (2006). *Assessing and managing violence risk in juveniles.* New York: Guilford Press.

Brennan, P. A., Mednick, S. A., & Hidgins, S. (2000). Major mental disorders and criminal violence in a Danish birth cohort. *Archives of General Psychiatry, 57,* 494–500.

Brodsky, S. L. (1991). *Testifying in court: Guidelines and maxims for the expert witness.* Washington, DC: American Psychological Association.

Brodsky, S. L. (1999). *The expert expert witness: More maxims and guidelines for testifying in court.* Washington, DC: American Psychological Association.

Brodsky, S. L. (2004). *Coping with cross-examination and other pathways to effective testimony.* Washington, DC: American Psychological Association.

Brown, S. L., St. Amand, M. D., & Zamble, E. (2009). The dynamic prediction of criminal recidivism: A three-wave prospective study. *Law and Human Behavior, 33,* 25–45.

Burt, M. R. (1980). Cultural myths and supports for rape. *Journal of Personality and Social Psychology, 38,* 217–230.

Campbell, J. C. (1986). Assessment of risk of homicide for battered women. *Advances in Nursing Science, 8,* 36–51.

Campbell, J. C. (1995). Prediction of homicide of and by battered women. In J. C. Campbell (Ed.), *Assessing dangerousness: Violence by sexual offenders, batterers, and child abusers* (pp. 96–113). Thousand Oaks, CA: Sage.

Campbell, T. W. (2000). Sexual predator evaluations and phrenology: Considering issues of evidentiary reliability. *Behavioral Sciences and the Law, 18,* 111–130.

Campbell, T. W. (2003). Sex offenders and actuarial risk assessment: Ethical considerations. *Behavioral Sciences and the Law, 21,* 269–279.

Carson, D. (2008). Editorial: Justifying risk decisions. *Criminal Behaviour and Mental Health, 18,* 139–144.

Cattaneo, L. B., & Goodman, L. A. (2005). Risk factors for reabuse in intimate partner violence: A cross-disciplinary critical review. *Trauma, Violence, and Abuse, 6,* 141–175.

Caudill, O. B., Jr. (2002). Risk management for psychotherapists: Avoiding the pitfalls. In L. VandeCreek & T. L. Jackson (Eds.), *Innovations in clinical practice: A source book* (Vol. 20, pp. 307–323). Sarasota, FL: Professional Resource Press.

Check, J. V. P. (1985). *The Hostility Towards Women Scale.* Doctoral dissertation, University of Manitoba.

Chess, C., Salomone, K. L., & Hance, B. J. (1995). Improving risk communication in government: Research priorities. *Risk Analysis, 15,* 127–135.

Cheston, J., Mills, J. F., & Kroner, D. G. (2007, June). *The two-tiered violence risk estimates: Preliminary validity of a dynamic–actuarial approach to measuring and managing violence risk.* Poster session presented at the North American Correctional and Criminal Justice Psychology Conference, Ottawa, Canada.

Cleckley, H. (1959). Psychopathic states. In S. Arieti (Ed.), *American handbook of psychiatry* (Vol. 1, pp. 567–588). New York: Basic Books.

Cleckley, H. (1976). *The mask of sanity.* St. Louis: Mosby.

Coid, J. (1993). Current concepts and classifications of psychopathic disorder. In P. Tyrer & G. Stein (Eds.), *Personality disorder reviewed* (pp. 113–164). London: Gaskell.

Committee on Ethical Guidelines for Forensic Psychology (1991). Specialty guidelines for forensic psychologists. *Law and Human Behavior, 15*, 655–665.

Conroy, M. A. (2003). Evaluation of sexual predators. In A. Goldstein (Ed.), *Forensic psychology* (pp. 463–484). Hoboken, NJ: Wiley.

Cooke, D. J., & Michie, C. (2001). Refining the construct of psychopathy: Towards a hierarchical model. *Psychological Assessment, 13*, 171–188.

Cooke, D. J., Michie, C., & Skeem, J. (2007). Understanding the structure of the Psychopathy Checklist—Revised: An exploration of methodological confusion. *British Journal of Psychiatry, 190*, s39–s50.

Coulson, G., Ilacqua, G., Nutbrown, V., Giulekas, D., & Cudjoe, F. (1996). Predictive utility of the LSI for incarcerated female offenders. *Criminal Justice and Behavior, 23*, 427–439.

Craig, L. A., Beech, A., & Browne, K. D. (2006). Cross-validation of the Risk Matrix 2000 sexual and violent scales. *Journal of Interpersonal Violence, 21*, 612–633.

Crowne, D. P., & Marlowe, D. (1960). A new scale of social desirability independent of psychopathology. *Journal of Consulting Psychology, 24*, 349–354.

Cuffel, B. J., Shumway, M., Choulijian, T. L., & MacDonald, T. (1994). A longitudinal study of substance use and community violence in schizophrenia. *Journal of Nervous and Mental Disease, 182*, 704–708.

Culhane, D. P., Averyt, J., & Hadley, T. R. (1998). The prevalence of treated behavioral disorders among adult shelter users. *American Journal of Orthopsychiatry, 26*, 207–232.

Dahle, K. P. (2006). Strengths and limitations of actuarial prediction of criminal reoffence in a German prison sample: A comparative Study of LSI-R, HCR-20, and PCL-R. *International Journal of Law and Psychiatry, 29*, 431–442.

Daubert v. Merrell Dow Pharmaceuticals, Inc., 113S. Ct. 2786 (1993).

Dawes, R. M. (1999). A message from psychologists to economists: Mere predictability doesn't matter like it should (without a good story appended to it). *Journal of Economic Behavior and Organization, 39*, 29–40.

Dawes, R. M., Faust, D., & Meehl, P. E. (1989). Clinical versus actuarial judgment. *Science, 243*, 1668–1673.

Dean, K., Walsh, E., Moran, P., Tyrer, P., Creed, F., Byford, S., et al. (2006). Violence in women with psychosis. *British Journal of Psychiatry, 188*, 264–270.

Dempster, R. J., & Hart, S. D. (2002). The relative utility of fixed and variable risk factors in discriminating sexual recidivists and nonrecidivists. *Sexual Abuse: A Journal of Research and Treatment, 14*, 121–138.

Descutner, C. J., & Thelen, M. H. (1991). Development and validation of a Fear-of-Intimacy Scale. *Psychological Assessment: A Journal of Consulting and Clinical Psychology, 3*, 218–225.

de Vogel, V., & de Ruiter, C. (2004). Differences between clinicians and researchers in assessing risk of violence in forensic psychiatric patients. *Journal of Forensic Psychiatry and Psychology, 15*, 145–164.

de Vogel, V., & de Ruiter, C. (2005). The HCR-20 in personality disordered female offenders: A comparison with matched sample of males. *Clinical Psychology and Psychotherapy, 12*, 226–240.

de Vogel, V., de Ruiter, C., van Beek, D., & Mead, G. (2004). Predictive validity of the SVR-20 and Static-99 in a Dutch sample of treated sex offenders. *Law and Human Behavior, 28,* 235–251.

Dolan, M., & Khawaja, A. (2004). The HCR-20 and post-discharge outcome in male patients discharged from medium security in the UK. *Aggressive Behavior, 30,* 469–483.

Doren, D. M. (2004). Stability of the interpretive risk percentages for the RRA-SOR and Static-99. *Sexual Abuse: A Journal of Research and Treatment, 16,* 25–36.

Doyle v. United States, 530 F. Sup. 1278 (D.C. Cal. 1982).

Doyle, M., & Dolan, M. (2002). Violence risk assessment: Combining actuarial and clinical information to structure clinical judgments for the formulation and management of risk. *Journal of Psychiatric and Mental Health Nursing, 9,* 649–657.

Douglas, K. S., & Kropp, P. R. (2002). A prevention-based paradigm for violence risk assessment: Clinical and research applications. *Criminal Justice and Behavior, 29,* 617–658.

Douglas, K. S., & Ogloff, J. R. P. (2003). The impact of confidence on the accuracy of structured professional and actuarial violence risk judgments in a sample of forensic psychiatric patients. *Law and Human Behavior, 27,* 573–587.

Douglas, K. S., Ogloff, J. R. P., Nicholls, T. L., & Grant, I. (1999). Assessing risk for violence among psychiatric patients: The HCR-20 Violence Risk Assessment Scheme and the Psychopathy Checklist: Screening version. *Journal of Consulting and Clinical Psychology, 67,* 917–930.

Douglas, K. S., & Webster, C. D. (1999). The HCR-20 Violence Risk Assessment Scheme: Concurrent validity in a sample of incarcerated offenders. *Criminal Justice and Behavior, 26,* 3–19.

Douglas, K. S., Yeomans, M., & Boer, D. P. (2005). Comparative validity analysis of multiple measures of violence risk in a sample of criminal offenders. *Criminal Justice and Behavior, 32,* 479–510.

Dowden, C., & Andrews, D.A. (1999). What works for female offenders: A meta-analytic review. *Crime and Delinquency, 45,* 438–452.

Draine, J., Salzer, M. S., Culhane, D. P., & Hadley, T. R. (2002). Role of social disadvantage in crime, joblessness, and homelessness among persons with serious mental illness. *Psychiatric Services, 53,* 565–573.

Drake, R. E., Wallach, M. A., & McGovern, M. P. (2005). Future directions in preventing relapse to substance abuse among clients with severe mental illnesses. *Psychiatric Services, 56,* 1297–1302.

Ducro, C., & Pham, T. (2006). Evaluation of the SORAG and the Static-99 on Belgian sex offenders committed to a forensic facility. *Sexual Abuse: A Journal of Research and Treatment, 18,* 15–26.

Dvoskin, J. A., & Heilbrun, K. (2001). Risk assessment and release decision-making: Toward resolving the great debate. *Journal of the American Academy of Psychiatry and the Law, 29,* 6–10.

Edens, J. F. (2001). Misuses of the Hare Psychopathy Checklist—Revised in court: Two case examples. *Journal of Interpersonal Violence, 16,* 1082–1093.

Edens, J. F. (2006). Unresolved controversies concerning psychopathy: Implication for clinical and forensic decision making. *Professional Psychology: Research and Practice, 37, 69–65.*

Edens, J. F., Buffington-Vollum, J. K., Keilen, A., Roskamp, P., & Anthony, C. (2005). Predictions of future dangerousness in capital murder trials: Is it time to "disinvent the wheel"? *Law and Human Behavior, 29, 55–86.*

Edens, J. F., & Campbell, J. S. (2007). Identifying youths at risk for institutional misconduct: A meta-analytic investigation of the Psychopathy Checklist measures. *Psychological Services, 4, 13–27.*

Edens, J. F., Campbell, J. S., & Weir, J. M. (2007).Youth psychopathy and criminal recidivism: A meta-analysis of the psychopathy checklist measures. *Law and Human Behavior, 31, 53–75.*

Edens, J. F., Colwell, L. H., Desforges, D. M., & Fernandez, K. (2005). The impact of mental health evidence on support for capital punishment: Are defendants labeled psychopathic considered more deserving of death? *Behavioral Sciences and the Law, 23, 603–625.*

Edens, J. F., Guy, L. S., & Fernandez, K. (2003). Psychopathic traits predict attitudes toward a juvenile capital murderer. *Behavioral Sciences and the Law, 21, 807–828.*

Edens, J. F., Marcus, D. K., Lilienfeld, S. O., & Poythress, N. G. (2006). Psychopathic, not psychopathic: Taxometric evidence for the dimensional structure of psychopathy. *Journal of Abnormal Behavior, 115, 131–144.*

Edens, J. F., Skeem, J. L., & Douglas, K. S. (2006). Incremental validity analysis of the Violence Risk Appraisal Guide and the Psychopathy Checklist: Screening Version in a civil psychiatric sample. *Assessment, 13, 368–374.*

Einhorn, H. J. (1986). Accepting error to make less error. *Journal of Personality Assessment, 50, 387–395.*

Endrass, J., Urbaniok, F., Held, L., Vetter, S., & Rossegger, A. (2008). Accuracy of the Static-99 in predicting recidivism in Switzerland. *International Journal of Offender Therapy and Comparative Criminology, 53, 482–490.*

Fass, T. L., Heilbrun, K., Dematteo, D., & Fretz, R. (2008). The LSI-R and the COMPAS: Validation data on two risk-need tools. *Criminal Justice and Behavior, 35, 1095–1108.*

Fed. R. Evid. 702 (2000).

Feder, L. (1994). Psychiatric hospitalization history and parole decisions. *Law and Human Behavior, 18, 395–410.*

Flores, A. W., Lowenkamp, C. T., Holsinger, A. M., & Latessa, E. J. (2006). Predicting outcome with the Level of Service Inventory—Revised: The importance of implementation integrity. *Journal of Criminal Justice, 34, 523–529.*

Folsom, J., & Atkinson, J. L. (2007). The generalizability of the LSI-R and the CAT to the prediction of recidivism in female offenders. *Criminal Justice and Behavior, 34, 1044–1056.*

Forth, A. E., Kosson, D. S., & Hare, R. D. (2003). Hare Psychopathy Checklist: Youth Version (PCL:YV). Toronto: Multi-Health Systems.

Fujii, D. E. M., Tokioka, A. B., Lichton, A. I., & Hishinuma, E. (2005). Ethnic differences in prediction of violence risk with the HCR-20 among psychiatric inpatients. *Psychiatric Services, 56, 711–716.*

Gacono, C. B. (2000). Suggestions for implementation and use of the psychopathy checklists in forensic and clinical practice. In C. B. Gacono (Ed.), *The clinical and forensic assessment of psychopathy: A practitioner's guide* (pp. 175–201). Mahwah, NJ: Erlbaum.

Gambrill, E. D., & Richey, C. A. (1975). An assertion inventory for use in assessment and research. *Behavior Therapy, 6,* 550–561.

Gellerman, D. M., & Suddath, R. (2005).Violent fantasy, dangerousness, and the duty to warn and protect. *Journal of the American Academy of Psychiatry and the Law, 33,* 484–495.

Gendreau, P., Goggin, C., French, S., & Smith, P. (2006). Practicing psychology in correctional settings. In I. Weiner & A. Hess (Eds.), *The handbook of forensic psychology* (3rd ed., pp. 722–750). Hoboken, NJ: Wiley.

Gendreau, P., Goggin, C., & Smith, P. (2002). Is the PCL-R really the "unparalleled" measure of offender risk?: A lesson in knowledge cumulation. *Criminal Justice and Behavior, 29,* 397–426.

Gendreau, P., Little, T., & Goggin, C. (1996). A meta-analysis of the predictors of adult offender recidivism: What works! *Criminology, 34,* 575–607.

Girard, L., & Wormith, J. S. (2004). The predictive validity of the Level of Service Inventory—Ontario Revision on general and violent recidivism among various offender groups. *Criminal Justice and Behavior, 31,* 150–181.

Glover, A. J. J., Nicholson, D. E., Hemmati, T., Bernfeld, G. A., & Quinsey, V. L. (2002). A comparison of predictors of general and violent recidivism among high-risk federal offenders. *Criminal Justice and Behavior, 29,* 235–249.

Goldstein, A. M. (2006). Overview of forensic psychology. In A. M. Goldstein & I. B. Weiner (Eds.), *Handbook of psychology: Vol. 11. Forensic psychology* (pp. 3–20). Hoboken, NJ: Wiley.

Good, M.I. (1978). Primary affective disorder, aggression, and criminality. *Archives of General Psychiatry, 35,* 954–960.

Goodman, L. A., Dutton, M. A., & Bennett, L. (2000). Predicting repeat abuse among arrested batterers: Use of the Danger Assessment Scale in the criminal justice system. *Journal of Interpersonal Violence, 15,* 63–74.

Grann, M., Belfrage, H., & Tengstrom, A. (2000). Actuarial assessment of risk for violence: Predictive validity of the VRAG and the historical part of the HCR-20. *Criminal Justice and Behavior, 27,* 97–114.

Grann, M., & Langstrom, N. (2007). Actuarial assessment of violence risk: To weigh or not to weigh. *Criminal Justice and Behavior, 34,* 22–36.

Grann, M., & Wedin, I. (2002). Risk factors for recidivism among spousal assault and spousal homicide offenders. *Psychology, Crime and Law, 8,* 5–23.

Gray, N. S., Fitzgerald, S., Taylor, J., MacCulloch, M. J., & Snowden, R. J. (2007). Predicting future reconviction in offenders with intellectual disabilities: The predictive efficacy of VRAG, PCL-SV, and the HCR-20. *Psychological Assessment, 19,* 474–479.

Gray, N.S., Hill, C., McGleish, A., Timmons, D., MacCulloch, M.J., & Snowden, R. J. (2003). Prediction of violence and self-harm in mentally disordered offenders: A prospective study of the efficacy of HCR-20, PCL-R, and psychiatric symptomatology. *Journal of Consulting and Clinical Psychology, 71,* 443–451.

Gray, N. S., Snowden, R. J., MacCulloch, S., Phillips, H., Taylor, J., & MacCulloch, M. J. (2004). Relative efficacy of criminological, clinical, and personality measures of future risk of offending in mentally disordered offenders: A comparative study of the HCR-20, PCL:SV, and OGRS. *Journal of Consulting and Clinical Psychology, 72,* 523–530.

Green, D. M., & Swets, J. A. (1966). *Signal detection theory and psychophysics.* New York: Wiley.

Gretton, H. M., McBride, M., Hare, R. D., O'Shaughnessy, R., & Kumka, G. (2001). Psychopathy and recidivism in adolescent sex offenders. *Criminal Justice and Behavior, 28,* 427–449.

Grove, W. M., & Meehl, P. E. (1996). Comparative efficiency of informal (subjective, impressionistic) and formal (mechanical, algorithmic) prediction procedures: The clinical–statistical controversy. *Psychology, Public Policy, and Law, 2,* 293–323.

Grubin, D. (1998). *Sex offending against children: Understanding the risk* (Police Research Series Paper 99). London: Home Office.

Guay, J. P., Ruscio, J., Knight, R. A., & Hare, R. D. (2007). A taxometric analysis of the latent structure of psychopathy: Evidence for dimensionality. *Journal of Abnormal Psychology, 116,* 701–716.

Guy, L. S., Edens, J. F., Anthony, C., & Douglas, K. S. (2005). Does psychopathy predict institutional misconduct among adults?: A meta-analytic investigation. *Journal of Consulting and Clinical Psychology, 73,* 1056–1064.

Hanson, R. K. (1997). *The development of a brief actuarial risk scale for sexual offence recidivism* (User Report 97-04). Ottawa: Department of the Solicitor General of Canada.

Hanson, R. K. (1998). What do we know about sex offender risk assessment? *Psychology, Public Policy, and Law, 4,* 50–72.

Hanson, R. K. (2006). Does Static-99 predict recidivism among older sexual offenders? *Sex Abuse, 18,* 343–355.

Hanson, R. K., & Bussiere, M. T. (1998). Predicting relapse: A meta-analysis of sexual offender recidivism studies. *Journal of Consulting and Clinical Psychology, 66,* 348–362.

Hanson, R. K., & Harris, A. J. R. (2000). Where should we intervene?: Dynamic predictors of sex offense recidivism. *Criminal Justice and Behavior, 27,* 6–35.

Hanson, R. K., & Harris, A. J. R. (2001). A structured approach to evaluating change among sexual offenders. *Sexual Abuse: A Journal of Research and Treatment, 13,* 105–122.

Hanson, R. K., Harris, A. J. R., Scott, T., & Helmus, L. (2007). *Assessing the risk of sexual offenders on community supervision: The Dynamic Supervision Project* (Corrections User Report No. 2007-05). Ottawa: Public Safety Canada.

Hanson, R. K., Helmus, L., & Bourgon, G. (2007). *The validity of risk assessments for intimate partner violence: A meta-analysis* (Corrections User Report No. 2007-07). Ottawa: Public Safety Canada.

Hanson, R. K., & Morton-Bourgon, K. E. (2005). The characteristics of persistent sexual offenders: A meta-analysis of recidivism studies. *Journal of Consulting and Clinical Psychology, 73,* 1154–1163.

Hanson, R. K., & Morton-Bourgon, K. E. (2007). *The accuracy of recidivism risk assessment for sexual offenders: A meta-analysis* (Corrections User Report No. 2007-01). Ottawa: Public Safety Canada.

Hanson, R. K., & Morton-Bourgon, K. E. (2009). The accuracy of recidivism risk assessments for sexual offenders: A meta-analysis of 118 studies. *Psychological Assessment, 21,* 1–21.

Hanson, R. K., & Thornton, D. (2000). Improving risk assessments for sex offenders: A comparison of three actuarial scales. *Law and Human Behavior, 24,* 119–136.

Hanson, R. K., & Thornton, D. (2003). *Notes on the development of the Static-2002* (User Report 2003-01). Ottawa: Public Safety Canada.

Hanson, R. K., & Wallace-Capretta, S. (2004). Predictors of criminal recidivism among male batterers. *Psychology, Crime, and Law, 10,* 413–427.

Hare, R. D. (1965). Temporal gradient of fear arousal in psychopaths. *Journal of Abnormal Psychology, 70,* 442–445.

Hare, R. D. (1968). Detection threshold for electric shock in psychopaths. *Journal of Abnormal Psychology, 73,* 268–272.

Hare, R. D. (1978). Psychopathy and electrodermal responses to nonsignal stimulation. *Biological Psychology, 6,* 237–246.

Hare, R. D. (1980). A research scale for the assessment of psychopathy in criminal populations. *Personality and Individual Differences, 1,* 111–119.

Hare, R. D. (1982). Psychopathy and the personality dimensions of psychoticism, extraversion, and neuroticism. *Personality and Individual Differences, 3,* 35–42.

Hare, R. D. (1984). Performance of psychopaths on cognitive tasks related to frontal lobe function. *Journal of Abnormal Psychology, 93,* 133–140.

Hare, R. D. (1985). Comparison of procedures for the assessment of psychopathy. *Journal of Consulting and Clinical Psychology, 53,* 7–16.

Hare, R. D. (1991). *The Hare Psychopathy Checklist—Revised (Manual).* Toronto: Multi-Health Systems.

Hare, R. D. (1996). Psychopathy: A clinical construct whose time has come. *Criminal Justice and Behavior, 23,* 25–54.

Hare, R. D. (2003). *The Hare Psychopathy Checklist—Revised* (PCL-R, 2nd ed.). Toronto: Multi-Health Systems.

Hare, R. D., & Forth, A. E. (1985). Psychopathy and lateral preference. *Journal of Abnormal Psychology, 94,* 541–546.

Hare, R. D., Harpur, T. J., Hakistian, A. R., Forth, A. E., & Hart, S. D. (1990). The revised Psychopathy Checklist: Reliability and factor structure. *Psychological Assessment: A Journal of Consulting and Clinical Psychology, 2,* 338–341.

Hare, R. D., Hart, S. D., & Harpur, T. J. (1991). Psychopathy and the DSM-IV criteria for antisocial personality disorder. *Journal of Abnormal Behavior, 100,* 391–398.

Hare, R. D., & McPherson, L. M. (1984). Violent and aggressive behavior by criminal psychopaths. *International Journal of Law and Psychiatry, 7,* 35–50.

Harris, A. J. R., & Hanson, R. K. (2004). *Sex offender recidivism: A simple question* (Public Safety User Report No. 2004-03). Ottawa: Public Safety Canada.

Harris, A. J. R., Phenix, A., Hanson, R. K., & Thornton, D. (2007). *Static-99 coding rules revised—2003* (Corrections User Report No. 2003-03). Ottawa: Public Safety Canada.

Harris, G. T., & Rice, M. E. (2003). Actuarial assessment of risk among sex offenders. *Annals of the New York Academy of Science, 989,* 198–210.

Harris, G. T., & Rice, M. E. (2007a). Adjusting actuarial violence risk assessments based on aging or the passage of time. *Criminal Justice and Behavior, 34,* 297–313.

Harris, G. T., & Rice, M. E. (2007b). Characterizing the value of actuarial violence risk assessments. *Criminal Justice and Behavior, 34,* 1638–1658.

Harris, G. T., Rice, M. E., & Camilleri, J. A. (2004). Applying a forensic actuarial assessment (the Violence Risk Appraisal Guide) to nonforensic patients. *Journal of Interpersonal Violence, 19,* 1063–1074.

Harris, G. T., Rice, M. E., & Cormier, C. A. (2002). Prospective replication of the Violence Risk Appraisal Guide in predicting violent recidivism among forensic patients. *Law and Human Behavior, 26,* 377–394.

Harris, G. T., Rice, M. E., & Quinsey, V. L. (1993). Violent recidivism of mentally disordered offenders: The development of a statistical prediction instrument. *Criminal Justice and Behavior, 20,* 315–335.

Harris, G. T., Rice, M. E., & Quinsey, V. L. (1994). Psychopathy as a taxon: Evidence that psychopathys are a discrete class. *Journal of Consulting and Clinical Psychology, 62,* 387–397.

Harris, G. T., Rice, M. E., Quinsey, V. L., Lalumiere, M. L., Boer, D., & Lang, C. (2003). A multisite comparison of actuarial risk instruments for sex offenders. *Psychological Assessment, 15,* 413–425.

Harris, G. T., Skilling, T., & Rice, M. E. (2001). The construct of psychopathy. *Crime and Justice, 28,* 197–264.

Hart, H. (1923). Predicting parole success. *Journal of Criminal Law, Criminology and Police Science, 14,* 405–413.

Hart, S. D. (1998a). Psychopathy and the risk for violence. In D. J. Cooke, A. E. Forth, & R. D. Hare (Eds.), *Psychopathy: Theory, research, and implications for society* (pp. 355–374). Dordrecht, The Netherlands: Kluwer Academic.

Hart, S. D. (1998b). The role of psychopathy in assessing risk for violence: Conceptual and methodological issues. *Legal and Criminological Psychology, 3,* 121–137.

Hart, S. D., Cox, D. N., & Hare, R. D. (1995). *Hare Psychopathy Checklist: Screening Version (PCL:SV).* Toronto: Multi-Health Systems.

Hart, S. D., & Hare, R. D. (1989). Discriminant validity of the Psychopathy Checklist in a forensic psychiatric population. *Psychological Assessment: A Journal of Consulting and Clinical Psychology, 1,* 211–218.

Hart, S. D., Hare, R. D., & Forth, A. E. (1994). Psychopathy as a risk marker for violence: Development and validation of a screening version of the revised Psychopathy Checklist. In J. Monahan & H. J. Steadman (Eds.), *Violence and mental disorders: Developments in risk assessment* (pp. 81–98). Chicago: University of Chicago Press.

Hart, S. D., Hare, R. D., & Harpur, T. J. (1992). The Psychopathy Checklist—Revised: An overview for researchers and clinicians. In J. Rosen & P. McReynolds (Eds.), *Advances in psychological assessment* (Vol. 7, pp. 103–130). New York: Plenum Press.

Hayes, L. M. (1995). Prison suicide: An overview and guide to prevention. *Prison Journal, 75,* 431–456.

Heckert, D. A., & Gondolf, E. W. (2004). Battered women's perceptions of risk versus risk factors and instruments in predicting repeat reassault. *Journal of Interpersonal Violence, 19,* 778–800.

Heilbrun, K. (1997). Prediction versus management models relevant to risk assessment: The importance of legal decision-making context. *Law and Human Behavior, 21,* 347–359.

Heilbrun, K. (2003). Violence risk: From prediction to management. In D. Carson & R. Bull (Eds.), *Handbook of psychology in legal contexts* (2nd ed., pp. 127–143). Hoboken, NJ: Wiley.

Heilbrun, K., Dvoskin, J., Hart, S., & McNiel, D. (1999). Violence risk communication: Implications for research, policy, and practice. *Health, Risk and Society, 1,* 91–106.

Heilbrun, K., Marczyk, G., Dematteo, D., & Mack-Allen, J. (2007). A principles-based approach to forensic mental health assessment: Utility and update. In A. M. Goldstein (Ed.), *Forensic psychology: Emerging topics and expanding roles* (pp. 45–72). Hoboken, NJ: Wiley.

Heilbrun, K., Nezu, C. M., Keeney, M., Chung, S., & Wasserman, A. L. (1998). Sexual offending: Linking assessment, intervention, and decision making. *Psychology, Public Policy, and Law, 4,* 138–174.

Heilbrun, K., O'Neill, M. L., Stevens, T. N., Strohman, L. K., Bowman, Q., & Lo, Y. L. (2004). Assessing normative approaches to communicating violence risk: A national survey of psychologists. *Behavioral Sciences and the Law, 22,* 187–196.

Heilbrun, K., O'Neill, M. L., Strohman, L. K., Bowman, Q., & Philipson, J. (2000). Expert approaches to communicating violence risk. *Law and Human Behavior, 24,* 137–148.

Heilbrun, K., Philipson, J., Berman, L., & Warren, J. (1999). Risk communication: Clincians' reported approaches and perceived values. *Journal of the American Academy of Psychiatry and the Law, 27,* 397–406.

Heltzel, T. (2007). Compatibility of therapeutic and forensic roles. *Professional Psychology: Research and Practice, 38,* 122–128.

Hemphill, J. F., & Hare, R. D., (2004). Some misconceptions about the Hare PCL-R and risk assessment: A reply to Gendreau, Goggin, and Smith. *Criminal Justice and Behavior, 31,* 203–243.

Hemphill, J. F., Hare, R. D., & Wong, S. (1998). Psychopathy and recidivism: A review. *Legal and Criminological Psychology, 3,* 139–170.

Hendricks, B., Werner, T., Shipway, L., & Turinetti, G. J. (2006). Recidivism among spousal abusers: Predictions and program evaluation. *Journal of Interpersonal Violence, 21,* 703–716.

Hess, A. K. (2006). Serving as an expert witness. In I. B. Weiner & A. K. Hess (Eds.), *The handbook for forensic psychology* (3rd ed.). Hoboken, NJ: Wiley.

Hiday, V. A. (2006). Putting community risk in perspective: A look at correlations, causes, and controls. *International Journal of Law and Psychiatry, 29,* 316–331.

Hilton, N. Z., Carter, A. M., Harris, G. T., & Sharpe, A. J. B. (2008). Does using nonnumerical terms to describe risk aid violence risk communication?: Clinician agreement and decision making. *Journal of Interpersonal Violence, 23,* 171–188.

Hilton, N. Z., & Harris, G. T. (2005). Predicting wife assault: A critical review and implications for policy and practice. *Trauma, Violence, and Abuse, 6,* 3–23.

Hilton, N. Z., & Harris, G. T. (2009). How nonrecidivism affects predictive accuracy: Evidence from a cross-validation of the Ontario Domestic Assault Risk Assessment (ODARA). *Journal of Interpersonal Violence, 24,* 326–337.

Hilton, N. Z., Harris, G. T., Rawson, K., & Beach, C. A. (2005). Communicating violence risk information to forensic decision makers. *Criminal Justice and Behavior, 32,* 97–116.

Hilton, N. Z., Harris, G. T., & Rice, M. E. (2001). Predicting violence by serious wife assaulters. *Journal of Interpersonal Violence, 16,* 408–423.

Hilton, N. Z., Harris, G. T., & Rice, M. E. (2006). Sixty-six years of research on the clinical versus actuarial prediction of violence. *Counseling Psychologist, 34,* 400–409.

Hilton, N. Z., Harris, G. T., & Rice, M. E. (2009). *Risk assessment for domestically violent men: Tools for criminal justice, offender intervention and victim services.* Washington, DC: American Psychological Association.

Hilton, N. Z., Harris, G. T., Rice, M. E., Houghton, R. E., & Eke, A. W. (2008). An indepth actuarial assessment for wife assault recidivism: The Domestic Violence Risk Appraisal Guide. *Law and Human Behavior, 32,* 150–163.

Hilton, N. Z., Harris, G. T., Rice, M. E., Lang, C., Cormier, C. A., & Lines, K. J. (2004). A brief actuarial assessment for the prediction of wife assault recidivism: The Ontario Domestic Assault Risk Assessment. *Psychological Assessment, 16,* 267–275.

Hilton, N. Z., & Simmons, J. L. (2001). The influence of actuarial risk assessment in clinical judgments and tribunal decision about mentally disordered offenders in maximum security. *Law and Human Behavior, 25,* 393–408.

Hodgins, S. (2007). Persistent violent offending: What do we know? *British Journal of Psychiatry, 190,* s12–s14.

Hodgins, S., & Cote, G. (1993). The Criminality of Mentally Disordered Offenders. *Criminal Justice and Behavior, 20,* 115–129.

Hollin, C. R., & Palmer, E. J. (2003). Level of Service Inventory—Revised profiles of violent and nonviolent prisoners. *Journal of Interpersonal Violence, 18,* 1075–1086.

Hollin, C. R., & Palmer, E. J. (2006). The Level of Service Inventory—Revised profile of English prisoners: Risk and reconviction analysis. *Criminal Justice and Behavior, 33,* 347–366.

Hollin, C. R., Palmer, E. J., & Clark, D. (2003). The Level of Service Inventory—Revised profile of English prisoners: A needs analysis. *Criminal Justice and Behavior, 30,* 422–440.

Holtfreter, K., & Cupp, R. (2007). Gender and risk assessment: The empirical status of the LSI-R for women. *Journal of Contemporary Criminal Justice, 23,* 363–382.

Howe, E. S. (1994). Judged person dangerousness as weighted averaging. *Journal of Applied Social Psychology, 24,* 1270–1290.

Hunter, R. H., Ritchie, A. J., & Spaulding, W. D. (2005). The Sell decision: Implications for psychological assessment and treatment. *Professional Psychology: Research and Practice, 36,* 467–475.

In the Matter of the Civil Commitment of G.G.N., 855 A.2d 569 (N.J. Ct. App. 2004).

Intrator, J., Hare, R. D., Stritzke, P., Brichtswein, K., Dorfman, D., Harpur, T., et al. (1997). A brain imaging (single photon emission computerized tomography) study of semantic and affective processing in psychopaths. *Biological Psychiatry, 42,* 96–103.

Jung, S., & Rawana, E. P. (1999). Risk and need assessment of juvenile offenders. *Criminal Justice and Behavior, 26,* 69–89.

Junginger, J., Claypoole, K., Laygo, R., & Crisanti, A. (2006). Effects of serious mental illness and substance abuse on criminal offenses. *Psychiatric Services, 57,* 879–882.

Kahneman, D., & Tversky, A. (1973). On the psychology of prediction. *Psychological Review, 80,* 237–251.

Kelly, C. E., & Welsh, W. N. (2008). The predictive validity of the Level of Service Inventory—Revised for drug-involved offenders. *Criminal Justice and Behavior, 35,* 819–831.

Kingston, D. A., Yates, P. M., Firestone, P., Babchishin, K., & Bradford, J. M. (2008). Long-term predictive validity of the Risk Matrix 2000: A comparison with the Static-99 and the Sex Offender Risk Appraisal Guide. *Sexual Abuse: A Journal of Research and Treatment, 20,* 466–484.

Knight, R. A., & Thornton, D. (2007). *Evaluating and improving assessment schemes for sexual recidivism: A long-term follow-up of convicted sexual offenders.* Washington, DC; U.S. Department of Justice.

Kosson, D. S., Steuerwald, B. L., Forth, A. E., & Kirkhart, K. J. (1997). A new method for assessing the interpersonal behavior of psychopathic individuals: Preliminary validation studies. *Psychological Assessment, 9,* 89–101.

Kroner, D. G., & Loza, W. (2001). Evidence for the efficacy of self-report in predicting nonviolent and violent criminal recidivism. *Journal of Interpersonal Violence, 16,* 168–177.

Kroner, D. G., & Mills, J. F. (2001). The accuracy of five risk appraisal instruments in predicting institutional misconduct and new convictions. *Criminal Justice and Behavior, 28,* 471–489.

Kroner, D. G., & Mills, J. F. (2002). *Criminal Attribution Inventory User Guide.* Kingston, ON: Author.

Kroner, D. G., Mills, J. F., & Morgan, R. D. (2007). Underreporting of crime-related content and the prediction of criminal recidivism among violent offenders. *Psychological Services, 4,* 85–95.

Kroner, D. G., Mills, J. F., & Reddon, J. R. (2005). A coffee can, factor analysis, and prediction of criminal risk: The structure of "criminality." *International Journal of Law and Psychiatry, 28,* 360–374

Kropp, P. R., & Hart, S. D. (2000). The Spousal Assault Risk Assessment (SARA) Guide: Reliability and validity in adult male offenders. *Law and Human Behavior, 24,* 101–118.

Kropp, P. R., Hart, S. D., & Lyon, D. R. (2002). Risk assessment of stalkers: Some problems and possible solutions. *Criminal Justice and Behavior, 29,* 590–616.

Kropp, P. R., Hart, S. D., Webster, C. D., & Eaves, D. (1994). *Manual for the Spousal Assault Risk Assessment Guide.* Vancouver: British Columbia Institute on Family Violence.

Kropp, P. R., Hart, S. D., Webster, C. D., & Eaves, D. (1995). *Manual for the Spousal Assault Risk Assessment Guide* (2nd ed.). Vancouver: British Columbia Institute on Family Violence.

Kropp, P. R., Hart, S. D., Webster, C. D., & Eaves, D. (1999). *Spousal Assault Risk Assessment: User's guide.* Toronto: Multi-Health Systems.

Lally, S. J. (2003). What tests are acceptable for use in forensic evaluations?: A survey of experts. *Professional Psychology: Research and Practice, 34,* 491–498.

Lalumiere, M. L., Harris, G. T., & Rice, M. E. (2001). Psychopathy and developmental instability. *Evolution and Human Behavior, 22,* 75–92.

Langton, C. M., Barbaree, H. E., Hansen, K. T., Harkins, L., & Peacock, E. J. (2007). Reliability and validity of the Static-2002 among adult sexual offenders with reference to treatment status. *Criminal Justice and Behavior, 34,* 616–640.

Langton, C. M., Barbaree, H. E., Seto, M. C., Peacock, E. J., Harkins, L., & Hansen, K. T. (2007). Actuarial assessment of risk for reoffense among adult sex offenders: Evaluating the predictive accuracy of the Static-2002 and five other instruments. *Criminal Justice and Behavior, 34,* 37–59.

Latessa, E. T., Cullen, F. T., & Gendreau, P. (2002). Beyond correctional quackery—Professionalism and the possibility of effective treatment. *Federal Probation, 66,* 43–50.

Lawson, J. S., Marshall, W. L., & McGrath, P. (1979). The Social Self-Esteem Inventory. *Educational and Psychological Measurement, 39,* 803–811.

Leistico, A. R., Salekin, R. T., DeCoster, J., & Rogers, R. (2008). A large-scale meta-analysis relating the Hare measures of psychopathy to antisocial conduct. *Law and Human Behavior, 32,* 28–45.

Link, B. G., Andrews, H., & Cullen, F. T. (1992). The violent and illegal behavior of mental patients reconsidered. *American Sociological Review, 57,* 275–292.

Link, B. G., Monahan, J., Stueve, A., & Cullen, F. T. (1999). Real in their consequences: A sociological approach to understanding the association between psychotic symptoms and violence. *American Sociological Review, 64,* 316–332.

Lipsey, M. W., & Cullen, F. T. (2007). The effectiveness of correctional rehabilitation: A review of systematic reviews. *Annual Review of Law and the Social Sciences, 3,* 297–320.

Looman, J., & Abracen, J. (2010). Comparison of measures of risk for recidivism in sexual offenders. *Journal of Interpersonal Violence, 25,* 791–807.

Lowenkamp, C. T., Holsinger, A. M., & Latessa, E. J. (2001). Risk/need assessment, offender classification, and the role of childhood abuse. *Criminal Justice and Behavior, 28,* 543–563.

Loza, W., & Simourd, D. J. (1994). Psychometric evaluation of the Level of Supervision Inventory (LSI) among male Canadian federal offenders. *Criminal Justice and Behavior, 21,* 468–480.

Loza, W., Villeneuve, D. B., & Loza-Fanous, A. (2002). Predictive validity of the

Violence Risk Appraisal Guide: A tool for assessing violent offenders' recidivism. *International Journal of Law and Psychiatry, 25*, 85–92.

MacKenzie, D. L. (2000). Evidence-based corrections: Identifying what works. *Crime & Delinquency, 46*, 547–471.

MacKenzie, D. L. (2001) Corrections and sentencing in the 21st century: Evidence-based corrections and sentencing. *Prison Journal, 81*, 299–312.

Manchak, S. M., Skeem, J. L., & Douglas, K. S. (2007). Utility of the Revised Level of Service Inventory (LSI-R) in predicting recidivism after long-term incarceration. *Law and Human Behavior, 32*, 477–488.

McGrath, R. E. (2003). Enhancing accuracy in oberservational test scoring: The comprehensive system as a case example. *Journal of Personality Assessment, 81*, 104–110.

McNiel, D.E., & Binder, R.L. (1995). Correlates of accuracy in the assessment of psychiatric inpatients' risk of violence. *American Journal of Psychiatry, 152*, 901–906.

McNiel, D. E., Eisner, J. P., & Binder, R. L. (2003). The relationship between aggressive attributional style and violence by psychiatric patients. *Journal of Consulting and Clinical Psychology, 71*, 399–403.

Meisel, A., Roth, L. H., & Lidz, C. W. (1977). Toward a model of the legal doctrine of informed consent. *American Journal of Psychiatry, 134*, 285–289.

Melton, G. B., Petrila, J., Poythress, N. G., Slobogin, C., Lyons, P. M., Jr., Otto, R. K. (2007). *Psychological evaluation for the courts: A handbook for mental health professionals and lawyers* (3rd ed.). New York: Guilford Press.

Merriam-Webster's Collegiate Dictionary (10th ed.). (1999). Springfield, MA: Merriam-Webster Incorporated.

Mill, J., Caspi, A., Williams, B. S., Craig, I., Taylor, A., Polo-Tomas, M., et al. (2006). Prediction of heterogeneity in intelligence and adult prognosis by genetic polymorphisms in the dopamine system among children with attention-deficit/ hyperactivity disorder: Evidence from 2 birth cohorts. *Archives of General Psychiatry, 63*, 462–469.

Millon, T., Davis, R. D., & Millon, C. (1997). *Manual for the Millon Clinical Multiaxial Inventory—III* (2nd ed.). Minneapolis, MN: National Computer Systems.

Mills, J. F. (2005). Advances in the assessment and prediction of interpersonal violence. *Journal of Interpersonal Violence, 20*, 236–241.

Mills, J. F., Green, K., Kroner, D. G., & Morgan, T. (2010). *The perception and communication of criminal risk estimates.* Manuscript in preparation.

Mills, J. F., Jones, M. N., & Kroner, D. G. (2005). An examination of the generalizability of the LSI-R and VRAG probability bins. *Criminal Justice and Behavior, 32*, 565–585.

Mills, J. F., & Kroner, D. G. (1999). *Measures of criminal attitudes and associates user guide.* Kingston, ON: Authors.

Mills, J. F., & Kroner, D. G. (2005). *Two-tiered violence risk estimates.* Kingston, ON: Author.

Mills, J. F., & Kroner, D. G. (2006a). The effect of discordance among violence and general recidivism risk estimates on predictive accuracy. *Criminal Behaviour and Mental Health, 16*, 155–166.

Mills, J. F., & Kroner, D. G. (2006b). The effect of base-rate information on the perception of risk for re-offence. *American Journal of Forensic Psychology, 24,* 45–56.

Mills, J. F., & Kroner, D. G. (2006c). *The Associates for Success Group.* Unpublished treatment manual.

Mills, J. F., Kroner, D. G., & Forth, A. E. (2002). Measures of Criminal Attitudes and Associates (MCAA): Development, factor structure, reliability and validity. *Assessment, 9,* 240–253.

Mills, J. F., Kroner, D. G., & Hemmati, T. (2003). Predicting violence behavior through a static–stable variable lens. *Journal of Interpersonal Violence, 18,* 891–904.

Mills, J. F., Kroner, D. G., & Hemmati, T. (2004). The Measures of Criminal Attitudes and Associates (MCAA): The prediction of general and violent recidivism. *Criminal Justice and Behavior, 31,* 717–733.

Mills, J. F., Kroner, D. G., & Hemmati, T. (2007). The validity of violence risk estimates: An issue of item performance. *Psychological Services, 4,* 1–12.

Mills, J. F., Loza, W., & Kroner, D. G. (2003). Predictive validity despite social desirability: Evidence for the robustness of self-report among offenders. *Criminal Behaviour and Mental Health, 13,* 140–150.

Moffitt, T. E. (1993). The neuropsychology of conduct disorder. *Development and Psychopathology, 5,* 135–151.

Moffitt, T. E., Krueger, R. F., Caspi, A., & Fagan, J. (2000). Partner abuse and general crime: How are they the same? How are the different? *Criminology, 38,* 199–232.

Monahan, J. (1983). The prediction of violent behavior: Developments in psychology and law. In S. C. James & B. L. Hammonds (Eds.), *Psychology and the law* (Master Lecture Series, Vol. 2, pp. 151–176). Washington, DC: American Psychological Association.

Monahan, J. (1984). The prediction of violent behavior: Toward a second generation of theory and policy. *American Journal of Psychiatry, 141,* 10–15.

Monahan, J. (1996). Violence prediction: The past twenty and the next twenty years. *Criminal Justice and Behavior, 23,* 107–120.

Monahan, J., Heilbrun, K., Silver, E., Nabors, E., Bone, J., & Slovic, P. (2002). Communicating violence risk: Frequency formats, vivid outcomes, and forensic settings. *International Journal of Forensic Mental Health, 1,* 121–126.

Monahan, J., & Steadman, H. J. (1996). Violent storms and violent people: How meteorology can inform risk communication in mental health law. *American Psychologist, 51,* 931–938.

Monahan, J., Steadman, H. J., Silver, E., Appelbaum, P. S., Robbins, P. C., Mulvey, E. P., et al. (2001). *Rethinking risk assessment: The MacArthur Study of Mental Disorder and Violence.* New York: Oxford University Press.

Moore, M. E., & Hiday, V. A. (2006). Mental health court outcomes: A comparison of re-arrest and re-arrest severity between mental health court and traditional court participants. *Law and Human Behavior, 30,* 659–674.

Moracco, K., Runyan, C. W., & Butts, J. D. (1998). Femicide in North Carolina, 1920–1993: A statewide study of patterns and precursors. *Homicide Studies, 2,* 422–446.

Morey, L. C. (2007). *Personality Assessment Inventory manual.* Odessa, FL: Psychological Associates Resources.

Morgan, R. D., Rozycki, A. T., & Wilson, S. (2004). Inmate perceptions of mental health services. *Professional Psychology: Research and Practice, 35,* 389–396.

Morrison, D., & Gilbert, P. (2001). Social rank, shame and anger in primary and secondary psychopaths. *Journal of Forensic Psychiatry, 12,* 330–356.

Motiuk, L. L., Bonta, J., & Andrews, D. A. (1986). Classification in correctional halfway houses: The relative and incremental predictive validities of the Megargee-MMPI and LSI systems. *Criminal Justice and Behavior, 13,* 33–46.

Mullen, P. E., Burgess, P., Wallance, C., Palmer, S., & Ruschena, D. (2000). Community care and criminal offending in schizophrenia. *Lancet, 355,* 614–617.

Myers, K., & Winters, N. C. (2002). Ten-year review of rating scales. I: Overview of scale functioning, psychometric properties, and selection. *Journal of American Academy of Child Adolescent Psychiatry, 41,* 114–122.

Newman, J. P., & Schmitt, W. A. (1998). Passive avoidance in psychopathic offenders: A replication and extension. *Journal of Abnormal Psychology, 107,* 527–532.

Newman, J. P., Schmitt, W. A., & Voss, W. D. (1997). The impact of motivationally neutral cues on psychopathic individuals: Assessing the generality of the response modulation hypothesis. *Journal of Abnormal Psychology, 106,* 563–575.

Newman, J. P., Wallace, J. F., Schmitt, W. A., & Arnett, P. A. (1997). Behavioral inhibition system functioning in anxious, impulsive and psychopathic individuals. *Personality and Individual Differences, 23,* 583–592.

Nicholls, T. L., Ogloff, J. R. P., & Douglas, K. S. (2004). Assessing risk for violence among male and female civil psychiatric patients: The HCR-20, PCL:SV, and VSC. *Behavioral Sciences and the Law, 22,* 127–158.

Nicholson, R. A., & Norwood, S. (2000). The quality of forensic psychological assessments, reports, and testimony: Acknowledging the gap between promise and practice. *Law and Human Behavior, 24,* 9–44.

Northcraft, G. B., & Neale, M. A. (1987). Experts, amateurs, and real estate: An anchoring-and-adjustment perspective on property pricing decisions. *Organizational Behavior and Human Decision Processes, 39,* 84–97.

Nowicki, S., & Duke, M. P. (1983). The Nowicki–Strickland Life-Span Locus of Control Scales: Construct validation. In H. M. Lefcourt (Ed.), *Research with the locus of control construct: Vol. 2. Developments and social problems* (pp. 9–49). New York: Academic Press.

Nuffield, J. (1982). *Parole decision-making in Canada: Research towards decision guidelines.* Ottawa: Ministry of Supply and Services Canada.

Nugent, P. (2000). *The use of detention legislation: Factors affecting detention decisions and recidivism among high-risk federal offenders in Ontario.* Unpublished doctoral dissertation, Queens University, Ontario, Canada.

Olver, M. E., & Wong, S. C. P. (2006). Psychopathy, sexual deviance, and recidivism among sex offenders. *Sexual Abuse: A Journal of Research and Treatment, 18,* 65–82.

Olver, M. E., Wong, S. C. P., Nicholaichuk, T., & Gordon, A. (2007). The validity and reliability of the Violence Risk Scale—Sexual Offender Version: Assessing sex offender risk and evaluating therapeutic change. *Psychological Assessment, 19*, 318–329.

Ontario Ministry of the Solicitor General. (2000). *A guide to the Domestic Violence Supplementary Report form.* Toronto: Author.

Otto, R. K., & Heilbrun, K. (2002). The practice of forensic psychology: A look toward the future in light of the past. *American Psychologist, 57*, 5–18.

Packer, I. K. (2008). Specialized practice in forensic psychology: Opportunities and obstacles. *Professional Psychology: Research and Practice, 39*, 245–249.

Palmer, E. J., & Hollin, C. R. (2007). The Level of Service Inventory Revised with English women prisoners: A needs and reconviction analysis. *Criminal Justice and Behavior, 34*, 971–984.

Petrosino, A., Turpin-Petrosino, C., & Buehler, J. (2003). Scared Straight and other juvenile awareness programs for preventing juvenile delinquency: A systematic review of the randomized experimental evidence. *Annals of the American Academy of Political and Social Science, 589*, 41–62.

Pope, K. S. (2003). 10 fallacies in psychological assessment. Unpublished manuscript. Retrieved September 12, 2008, from *kspope.com/fallacies/assessment. php.*

Prochaska, J. O., & DiClemente, C. C. (1984). *The transtheoretical approach: Crossing traditional boundaries of therapy.* Homewood, IL: Dow–Jones–Irwin.

Prochaska, J. O., DiClemente, C. C., & Norcross, J. C. (1992). In search of how people change: Applications to addictive behaviors. *American Psychologist, 47*, 1102–1114.

Putkonen, H., Komulainen, E. J., Virkkunen, M., Eronen, M., & Lonnqvist, J. (2003). Risk of repeat offending among violent female offenders with psychotic and personality disorders. *American Journal of Psychiatry, 160*, 947–951.

Quattrocchi, M. R., & Schopp, R. F. (2005). TARASAURUS REX: A standard of care that could not adapt. *Psychology, Public Policy, and Law, 11*, 109–137.

Quinsey, V. L., Coleman, G., Jones, B., & Altrows, I. F. (1997). Proximal antecedents of eloping and reoffending among supervised mentally disordered offenders. *Journal of Interpersonal Violence, 12*, 794–813.

Quinsey, V. L., Book, A., & Skilling, T. A. (2004). A follow-up of deinstitutionalized men with intellectual disabilities and histories of antisocial behaviour. *Journal of Applied Research in Intellectual Disabilities, 17*, 243–253.

Quinsey, V. L., Skilling, T. A., Lalumiere, M. L., & Craig, W. M. (2004). *Juvenile delinquency: Understanding the origins of individual differences.* Washington, DC: American Psychological Association.

Quinsey, V. L., Harris, G. T., Rice, M. E., & Cormier, C. A. (1998). *Violent offenders: Appraising and managing risk.* Washington, DC: American Psychological Association.

Quinsey, V. L., Harris, G. T., Rice, M. E., & Cormier, C. A. (2006). *Violent offenders: Appraising and managing risk: 2nd edition.* Washington, DC: American Psychological Association.

Quinsey, V. L., Jones, G. B., Book, A. S., & Barr, K. N. (2006). The dynamic prediction of antisocial behavior among forensic psychiatric patients: A prospective field study. *Journal of Interpersonal Violence, 21*, 1539–1565.

Renn, O. (2004). Perception of risks. *Toxicology Letters, 149*, 405–413.

Rice, M. E., & Harris, G. T. (1995). Violent recidivism: Assessing predictive validity. *Journal of Consulting and Clinical Psychology, 63,* 737–748.

Rice, M. E., & Harris, G. T. (1997). Cross-validation and extension of the Violence Risk Appraisal Guide for Child Molesters and Rapists. *Law and Human Behavior, 21,* 231–241.

Rice, M. E., & Harris, G. T. (2003). The size and sign of treatment effects in sex offender therapy. *Annals of the New York Academy of Sciences, 989,* 428–440.

Rice, M. E., & Harris, G. T. (2005). Comparing effect sizes in follow-up studies: ROC Area, Cohen's d, and r. *Law and Human Behavior, 29,* 615–620.

Rice, M. E., Harris, G. T., & Cormier, C. (1992). Evaluation of a maximum security therapeutic community for psychopaths and other mentally disordered offenders. *Law and Human Behavior, 16,* 399–412.

Rice, M. E., Harris, G. T., & Quinsey, V. L. (1990). A follow-up of rapists assessed in a maximum-security psychiatric facility. *Journal of Interpersonal Violence, 5,* 435–448.

Rice, M. E., Harris, G. T., & Quinsey, V. L. (2002). The appraisal of violence risk. *Current Opinion in Psychiatry, 15,* 589–593.

Robbins, P. C., Monahan, J., & Silver, E. (2003). Mental disorder, violence, and gender. *Law and Human Behavior, 27,* 561–571.

Rogers, R. (2000). The uncritical acceptance of risk assessment in forensic practice. *Law and Human Behavior, 24,* 595–605.

Rogers, R., Salekin, R. T., & Sewell, K. W. (2000). The MCMI-III and the Daubert standard: Separating rhetoric from reality. *Law and Human Behavior, 24,* 501–506.

Rosen, G. M., & Davison, G. C. (2003). Psychology should list empirically supported principles of change (ESPs) and not credential trademarked therapies or other treatment packages. *Behavior Modification, 27,* 300–312.

Rosenfeld, B., & Harmon, R. (2002). Factors associated with violence in stalking and obsessional harassment cases. *Criminal Justice and Behavior, 29,* 671–691.

Roth, L. H., Meisel, A., & Lidz, C. W. (1977). Tests of competency to consent to treatment. *American Journal of Psychiatry, 134,* 279–284.

Rozycki-Lozano, A. T., Morgan, R. D., Murray, D. D., & Varghese, F. (in press). Prison tattoos as a reflection of the criminal lifestyle. *International Journal of Offender Therapy and Comparative Criminology.*

Russell, D., Peplau, L. A., & Cutrona, C. E. (1980). The revised UCLA Loneliness Scale. *Journal of Personality and Social Psychology, 39,* 472–480.

Salekin, R. T., Rogers, R., & Sewell, K. W. (1996). A review and meta-analysis of the Psychopathy Checklist and Psychopathy Checklist—Revised: Predictive validity of dangerousness. *Clinical Psychology: Science and Practice, 3,* 203–215.

Samra-Grewal, J., Pfeifer, J. E., & Ogloff, J. R. P. (2000). Recommendations for conditional release suitability: Cognitive biases and consistency in case management officers' decision-making. *Canadian Journal of Criminology, 42,* 421–447.

Sanderson, C. A., Zanna, A. S., & Darley, J. M. (2000). Making the punishment fit the crime and the criminal: Attributions of dangerousness as a mediator of liability. *Journal of Applied Social Psychology, 30,* 1137–1159.

Schlager, M. D., & Simourd, D. J. (2007). Validity of the Level of Service Inventory—Revised (LSI-R) among African-American and Hispanic male offenders. *Criminal Justice and Behavior, 34,* 545–554.

Schulsinger, F. (1972). Psychopathy: Heredity and environment. *International Journal of Mental Health, 1,* 190–206.

Schwalbe, C. (2004). Re-visioning risk assessment for human service decision making. *Children and Youth Services Review, 26,* 561–576.

Sell v. United States, 123 S. Ct. 512 (2002).

Serin, R. C. (1991). Psychopathy and violence in criminals. *Journal of Interpersonal Violence, 6,* 423–431.

Serin, R. C., & Amos, N. L. (1995). The role of psychopathy in the assessment of dangerousness. *International Journal of Law and Psychiatry, 18,* 231–238.

Shinn, M., Weitzman, B. C., Stojanovic, D., Knickman, J. R., Jimenez, L., Duchon, L., et al. (1998). Predictors of homelessness among families in New York City: From shelter request to housing stability. *American Journal of Public Health, 88,* 1651–1657.

Simourd, D. J. (1997). The Criminal Sentiments Scale—Modified and PID: Psychometric properties and construct validity of two measures of criminal attitudes. *Criminal Justice and Behavior, 24,* 52–70.

Simourd, D. J. (2004). Use of dynamic risk/need assessment instruments among long-term incarcerated offenders. *Criminal Justice and Behavior, 31,* 306–323.

Simourd, D. J., & Malcolm, P. B. (1998). Reliability and validity of the Level of Service Inventory—Revised among federally incarcerated sex offenders. *Journal of Interpersonal Violence, 13,* 261–274.

Sjostedt, G., & Langstrom, N. (2001). Actuarial assessment of sex offender recidivism risk: A cross-validation of the RRASOR and the Static-99 in Sweden. *Law and Human Behavior, 25,* 629–645.

Sjostedt, G., & Langstrom, N. (2002). Assessment of risk for criminal recidivism among rapists: A comparison of four different measures. *Psychology, Crime and Law, 8,* 25–40.

Skeem, J. L., & Cooke, D. (2010). Is criminal behavior a central component of psychopathy?: Conceptual directions for resolving the debate. *Psychological Assessment, 22,* 433–445.

Skeem, J. L., & Eno Louden, J. (2006). Toward evidence-based practice for probationers and parolees mandated for mental health treatment. *Psychiatric Services, 57,* 333–342.

Skeem, J. L., & Golding, S. L. (1998). Community examiners' evaluations of competence to stand trial: Common problems and suggestions for improvement. *Professional Psychology: Research and Practice, 29,* 357–367.

Skeem, J. L., Monahan, J., & Mulvey, E. P. (2002). Psychopathy, treatment involvement, and subsequent violence among civil psychiatric patients. *Law and Human Behavior, 26,* 577–603.

Skeem, J. L., Mulvey, E. P., Appelbaum, P., Banks, S., Grisso, T., Silver, E., et al. (2004). Identifying subtypes of civil psychiatric patients at high risk for violence. *Criminal Justice and Behavior, 31,* 392–437.

Skeem, J. L., Mulvey, E. P., & Lidz, C. W. (2000). Building mental health professionals' decisional models into tests of predictive validity: The accuracy of contextualized predictions of violence. *Law and Human Behavior, 24,* 607–628.

Skilling, T. A., Harris, G. T., Rice, M. E., & Quinsey, V. L. (2002). Identifying persistently antisocial offenders using the Hare Psychopathy Checklist and the DSM antisocial personality disorder criteria. *Psychological Assessment, 14,* 27–38.

Skilling, T. A., Quinsey, V. L., & Craig, W. M. (2001). Evidence of a taxon underlying serious antisocial behaviour in boys. *Criminal Justice and Behavior, 28,* 450–470.

Slovic, P. (1987). Perception of risk. *Science, 236,* 280–285.

Slovic, P., Fischhoff, B., & Lichtenstein, S. (1982). Facts and fears: Understanding perceived risk. In D. Kahneman, P. Slovic, & A. Tversky (Eds.), *Judgment under uncertainty* (pp. 463–489). New York: Cambridge University Press.

Slovic, P., Fischhoff, B., & Lichtenstein, S. (1984). Behavioral decision theory perspectives on risk and safety. *Acta Psychologica, 56,* 183–203.

Slovic, P., & Monahan, J. (1995). Probability, danger, and coercion: A study of risk perception and decision making in mental health law. *Law and Human Behavior, 19,* 49–65.

Slovic, P., Monahan, J., & MacGregor, D. G. (2000). Violence risk assessment and risk communication: The effects of using actual cases, providing instruction, and employing probability versus frequency formats. *Law and Human Behavior, 24,* 271–296.

Spielberger, C. D. (1983). *State–Trait Anxiety Inventory.* Palo Alto, CA: Consulting Psychologists.

Spielberger, C. D. (1988). *State–Trait Anger Expression Inventory professional manual.* Odessa, FL: Psychological Assessment Resources.

Stadtland, C., Hollweg, M., Kleindienst, N., Dietl, J., Reich, U., & Nedopil, N. (2005). Risk assessment and prediction of violent and sexual recidivism in sex offenders: Long-term predictive validity of four risk assessment instruments. *Journal of Forensic Psychiatry and Psychology, 16,* 92–108.

Stanley, B., & Galietta, M. (2006). Informed consent in treatment and research. In I. B. Weiner & A. K. Hess (Eds.), *The handbook for forensic psychology* (3rd ed., pp. 211–239). Hoboken, NJ: Wiley.

Steadman, H. J., Monahan, J., Appelbaum, P. S., Grisso, T., Mulvey, E. P., Roth, L. H., et al. (1994). *Designing a new generation of risk assessment research.* In J. Monahan & H. J. Steadman (Eds.), *Violence and mental disorder: Developments in risk assessment* (pp. 297–318). Chicago: University of Chicago Press.

Steadman, H. J., Mulvey, E. P., Monahan, J., Robbins, P. C., Appelbaum, P. S., Grisso, T. et al. (1998). Violence by people discharged from acute psychiatric inpatient facilities and by others in the same neighborhoods. *Archives of General Psychiatry, 55,* 393–401.

Straznickas, K. A., McNeil, D. N., & Binder, R. L. (1993). Violence toward family caregivers by mentally ill relatives. *Hospital and Community Psychiatry, 44,* 385–387.

Swanson, J., Estroff, S., Swartz, M., & Borom, R., (1997). Violence and severe mental disorder in clinical and community populations: The effects of psychotic symptoms, comorbidity, and lack of treatment. *Psychiatry: Interpersonal and Biological Processes, 60,* 1–22.

Swanson, J. W., Borum, R., Swartz, M. S., & Monahan, J. (1996). Psychotic symptoms and disorders and the risk of violent behaviour in the community. *Criminal Behaviour and Mental Health, 6,* 309–329.

Swanson, J. W., Holzer, C. E., Ganju, V. K., & Jono, R. T. (1990). Violence and psychiatric disorder in the community: Evidence from the Epidemiological Catchment Area Surveys. *Hospital and Community Psychiatry, 41,* 761–770.

Swanson, J. W., Swartz, M. S., Van Dorn, R. A., Elbogen, E. B., Wagner, H. R., Rosenheck, R. A., et al. (2006). A national study of violent behaviour in persons with schizophrenia. *Archives of General Psychiatry, 63,* 490–499.

Swartz, J. A., & Lurigio, A. J. (2007). Serious mental illness and arrest: The generalized mediating effect of substance use. *Crime and Delinquency, 53,* 581–604.

Swartz, M.S., Swanson, J. W., Hiday, V. A., Borum, R., Wagner, H. R., & Burns, B. J. (1998). Violence and severe mental illness: The effects of substance abuse and nonadherence to medication. *American Journal of Psychiatry, 155,* 226–231.

Swets, J. A. (1988). Measuring the accuracy of diagnostic systems. *Science, 240,* 1285–1293.

Tengström, A., Grann, M., Långström, N., & Kullgren, G. (2000). Psychopathy (PCL-R) as a predictor of violent recidivism among criminal offenders with schizophrenia. *Law and Human Behavior, 24,* 45–58.

Teplin, L. A., Abram, K. M., & McClelland, G. M. (1994). Does psychiatric disorder predict violent crime among released jail detainees? *American Psychologist, 49,* 335–342.

Thienhaus, O. J., & Piasecki, M. (1998). Assessment of psychiatric patients' risk of violence towards others. *Psychiatric Services, 49,* 1129–1147.

Thornton, D. (2002). Constructing and testing a framework for dynamic risk assessment. *Sexual Abuse: A Journal of Research and Treatment, 14,* 139–153.

Thornton, D. (2005). *Scoring guide for the Risk Matrix: 2000.5.* Unpublished manuscript.

Thornton, D., Mann, R., Webster, S., Blud, L., Travers, R., Friendship, C., et al. (2003). Distinguishing and combining risks for sexual and violent recidivism. In R. A. Prentky, E. S. Janus, & M. C. Seto (Eds.), *Sexually coercive behavior: Understanding and management* (Annals of the New York Academy of Sciences, Vol. 989, pp. 225–235). New York: New York Academy of Sciences.

Tolman, A. O., & Mullendore, K. B. (2003). Risk evaluations for the courts: Is service quality a function of specialization? *Professional Psychology, Research and Practice, 34,* 225–232.

Tolman, A. O., & Rhodes, J. (2005, March). *The admissibility of actuarial risk instruments in federal and state courts: Current status.* Paper presented at the annual conference of the American Psychology-Law Society, San Diego, CA.

Tolman, A. O., & Rotzien, A. L. (2007). Conducting risk evaluations for future violence: Ethical practice is possible. *Professional Psychology, Research and Practice, 38,* 71–79.

Villeneuve, D.B., & Quinsey, V.L. (1995). Predictors of general and violent recidivism among mentally disordered inmates. *Criminal Justice and Behavior, 22,* 397–410.

Wallace, C., Mullen, P. E., & Burgess, P. (2004). Criminal offending in schizophrenia over a 25–year period marked by deinstitutionalization and increasing prevalence of comorbid substance use disorders. *American Journal of Psychiatry, 161,* 716–727.

Wallsten, T. S., Budescu, D. V., Zwick, R., & Kemp, S. M. (1993). Preferences and reasons for communicating probabilistic information in verbal or numerical terms. *Bulletin of the Psychonomic Society, 31,* 135–138.

Walsh, E., Buchanan, A., & Fahy, T. (2002). Violence and schizophrenia: Examining the evidence. *British Journal of Psychiatry, 180,* 490–495.

Walsh, E., Gilvarry, C., Samele, C., Harvey, K., Manley, C., Tyrer, P., et al. (2001). Reducing violence in severe mental illness: Randomised controlled trial of intensive case management compared with standard care. *British Medical Journal, 323,* 1–5.

Walters, G. D. (2002). Developmental trajectories, transitions, and nonlinear dynamical systems: A model of crime deceleration and desistance. *International Journal of Offender Therapy and Comparative Criminology, 46,* 30–44.

Walters, G. D. (2003a). Predicting criminal justice outcomes with the Psychopathy Checklist and Lifestyle Criminality Screening Form: A meta-analytic comparison. *Behavioral Sciences and the Law, 21,* 89–102.

Walters, G. D. (2003b). Predicting institutional adjustment and recidivism with the Psychopathy Checklist factor scores: A meta-analysis. *Law and Human Behavior, 27,* 541–558.

Walters, G. D. (2006). Risk-appraisal versus self-report in the prediction of criminal justice outcomes: A meta-analysis. *Criminal Justice and Behavior, 33,* 279–304.

Walters, G. D. (2007). The latent structure of the criminal lifestyle: A taxometric analysis of the Lifestyle Criminality Screening Form and Psychological Inventory of Criminal Thinking Styles. *Criminal Justice and Behavior, 34,* 1623–1637.

Walters, G. D., Knight, R. A., Grann, M., & Dahle, K. P. (2008). Incremental validity of the Psychopathy Checklist facet scores: Predicting release outcome in six samples. *Journal of Abnormal Psychology, 117,* 396–405.

Walters, G. D., & White, T. W. (1989). The thinking criminal: A cognitive model of lifestyle criminality. *Criminal Justice Research Bulletin, 4,* 1–10.

Walters, G. D., White, T. W., & Denney, D. (1991). The Lifestyle Criminality Screening Form: Preliminary data. *Criminal Justice and Behavior, 18,* 406–418.

Warren, J. I., South, S. C., Burnette, M. L., Rogers, A., Friend, R., Bale, R., et al. (2005). *International Journal of Law and Psychiatry, 28,* 269–289.

Webster, C. D., Douglas, K. S., Eaves, C. D., & Hart, S. D. (1997). *The HCR-20 scheme: Assessing risk for violence: Version 2.* Vancouver: Mental Health, Law and Policy Institute, Simon Fraser University.

Webster, C. D., Eaves, D., Douglas, K. S., & Wintrup, A. (1995). *The HCR-20 scheme: The assessment of dangerousness and risk.* Vancouver: Simon Fraser University and British Columbia Forensic Psychiatric Services Commission.

Webster, C. D., Hucker, S. J., & Bloom, H. (2002). Transcending the actuarial versus clinical polemic in assessing risk for violence. *Criminal Justice and Behavior, 29,* 659–665.

Weisz, A. N., Tolman, R. M., & Saunders, D. G. (2000). Assessing the risk of severe domestic violence: The importance of survivor's predictions. *Journal of Interpersonal Violence, 15,* 75–90.

White v. United States, 401 U.S. 745 (1971).

Whiteacre, K. W. (2006). Testing the Level of Service Inventory—Revised (LSI-R) for racial/ethnic bias. *Criminal Justice Policy Review, 17,* 330–342.

Williams, K. R., & Houghton, A. B. (2004). Assessing the risk of domestic violence reoffending: A validation study. *Law and Human Behavior, 28,* 437–455.

Wilson, G. (1978). *The secrets of sexual fantasy.* London: Dent.

Wong, S. (1984). *The criminal and institutional behaviours of psychopaths* (Programs Branch User Report). Ottawa, Ontario: Ministry of the Solicitor General of Canada.

Wong, S. C. P., & Gordon, A. (2006). The validity and reliability of the Violence Risk Scale: A treatment friendly violence risk assessment tool. *Psychology, Public Policy, and Law, 12,* 279–309.

Wormith, J. S., & Goldstone, C. S. (1984). The clinical and statistical prediction of recidivism. *Criminal Justice and Behavior, 11,* 3–34.

Wright, E. M., Salisbury, E. J., & Van Voorhis, P. (2007). Predicting the prison misconducts of women offenders: The importance of gender-responsive needs. *Journal of Contemporary Criminal Justice, 23,* 310–340.

Zamble, E., & Quinsey, V. L. (1997). *The criminal recidivism process.* Cambridge, UK: Cambridge University Press.

Zinger, I., & Forth, A. E. (1998). Psychopathy and Canadian criminal proceedings: The potential for human rights abuses. *Canadian Journal of Criminology, 40,* 237–276.

Zumbo, B. D. (1999). The simple difference score as an inherently poor measure of change: Some reality, much mythology. In B. Thompson (Ed.), *Advances in social science methodology* (Vol. 4, pp. 269–304). Stamford, CT: JAI Press.

INDEX